MISCARRIAGE

MISCARRIAGE

MARGARET LEROY

ILLUSTRATED BY ANDREA NORTON

An OPTIMA book

© Margaret Leroy 1988

First published in 1988 by
Macdonald Optima, a division of
Macdonald & Co. (Publishers) Ltd

A BPCC PLC company

British Library Cataloguing in Publication Data

Leroy, Margaret
   Miscarriage.
   1. Miscarriage
   I. Title
   618.3′92   RG648

   ISBN 0-386-12888-1

Macdonald & Co. (Publishers) Ltd
3rd Floor
Greater London House
Hampstead Road
London NW1 7QX

Typeset by Leaper & Gard Ltd, Bristol
Printed and bound in Great Britain by
The Guernsey Press Co. Ltd.,
Channel Islands

CONTENTS

ACKNOWLEDGMENTS

I would like to thank the following people: Roy Farquharson (consultant gynaecologist, The Women's Hospital, Liverpool) for his careful reading of the manuscript and for his valuable comments on the medical material; Barbara Pickard (Honorary Research Fellow at the University of Leeds) who shared her extensive knowledge of nutrition with me; Caroline Bach and Madeleine Fullerton, who were thoughtful and sensitive in their response to the manuscript; Nigel Gray, who encouraged me to take on this project; my husband Michael for his love and patience, his perceptive comments and his excellent cooking; my daughter Rebecca for her forbearance with a mother who has been more than usually vague and preoccupied.

This book is the brainchild of Kathryn Ladley, who has worked formidably hard for the Miscarriage Association since she became secretary. Throughout the writing of this book I have enjoyed Kathryn's friendship and support, and we have had many stimulating discussions together. My understanding of miscarriage is grounded in what I have learnt from her.

Responsibility for the emphasis of the book, and for any errors, rests with me.

I am grateful for permission to quote from the following: *Your Reproductive Health At Risk*, by the General, Municipal, Boilermakers and Allied Trades Union; *VDUs and Pregnancy: a review of the evidence fo date* by the VDU Workers' Rights Campaign; 'Three Women' from *Winter Trees* by Sylvia Plath (Faber and Faber 1981); 'It Is My Fader Wyll' from *Medieval English Lyrics, a York Medieval Test,* edited by Theodore Silverstein (Edward Arnold 1971); 'With Child' from *Collected Poems 1918-1938* by Genevieve Taggard (Harper and Row Publishers Inc); *Out Loud* published by W.H. Allen.

INTRODUCTION

I have had two miscarriages, one at twelve weeks, the second at eight weeks. For years these were a hidden part of my life. I did not know anyone else who had miscarried, I had little idea about the causes of miscarriage, and I would have been very surprised to learn how frequently miscarriages occur. I scarcely talked about my experiences to anyone, and in this I was like many women who miscarry, for in our society miscarriage has been a secret aspect of women's experience.

Recently the silence about miscarriage has been broken a little. Much of the credit for this must go to the Miscarriage Association, a self-help organization founded in 1982 by a group of women, all of whom had suffered miscarriages. Every year, thousands of women contact the Association, looking for information and support. Kathryn Ladley, the secretary of the Association, felt that there was the potential for a book in the experiences of these women and the knowledge that the Association had amassed.

While researching for the book, I have read many hundreds of accounts of miscarriages. When there were specific questions in my mind, I have asked for help through the Miscarriage Association's newsletter, and I have been fortunate to receive many letters in response. I have talked to many women and men. Some interviews have been deliberately arranged, but at other times stories have been shared more casually, over coffee in friends' houses — for in any roomful of women there will be one who has suffered a miscarriage. I am tremendously grateful to all the women and men who broke the silence and shared their stories so generously with me.

1
MISCARRIAGE – WHAT HAPPENS

Miscarriage is 'the process by which the products of
conception are expelled from the uterus via the birth canal
before the 28th week of gestation.'
BEISCHER and MACKAY *Obstetrics and the Newborn*

Miscarriage is the worst thing that ever happened to me.
PAMELA JAMES

The broad medical definition of miscarriage covers a number of
different patterns. Some miscarriages take place very early in
pregnancy, before the woman even suspects she is pregnant.
This is a likely explanation for a period that is a little late and
heavier than usual. It has been suggested that nearly one in
three pregnancies end in this way.

The majority of reported miscarriages take place in the first
trimester, before 14 weeks of pregnancy. Quite often they
happen at 8 or 12 weeks, the times when the woman's period
would have been due if she was not pregnant. Perhaps one in six
confirmed pregnancies are lost before 14 weeks.

Only 3 per cent of miscarriages take place in the second
trimester, between 14 and 28 weeks of pregnancy. Sometimes
these miscarriages follow the same pattern of contractions and
bleeding as earlier miscarriages, but second trimester
miscarriages may also happen very quickly, with little pain or
bleeding. The dividing line between stillbirth and miscarriage is
based on the age at which a baby has some chance of surviving
once born. At present, the line is drawn at 28 weeks, but this
needs to be revised as babies born at 26 weeks now have a fair
chance of survival.

The 'missed miscarriage' is another possible pattern. In a
'missed miscarriage' the baby dies but is not expelled by the
uterus. The woman will probably stop feeling pregnant. There
may be a little bleeding now and then, and the uterus shrinks as
the amniotic fluid that surrounded the baby is re-absorbed.

This can happen at any stage of pregnancy. If the baby died early in pregnancy, a D & C (or scrape) will be done. If the baby died at a later stage, labour will be induced.

Once a woman has suffered three miscarriages, she is said to be suffering from recurrent or habitual miscarriage. Most doctors will not try to find out why a woman is miscarrying until it has happened three times. The justification for this is based on the statistics — statistically, you have as good a chance after your second miscarriage as after your first of having a successful pregnancy. However once you have had three miscarriages, the risk of your next pregnancy also ending in miscarriage goes up, although you still have a 50 per cent chance of a successful pregnancy. Even after four or more miscarriages, the chance that the next pregnancy will succeed is 40 per cent.[1]

No records are kept of miscarriage, so it is impossible to tell for certain how many women miscarry. However it has been estimated that in the region of 100,000 women suffer a miscarriage each year in the UK.

THREATENED MISCARRIAGE

Most miscarriages start with bleeding and with some kind of pain. The blood may be any shade from brown, indicating older blood, to bright red, meaning it is fresh. The pain is usually in the lower back, stomach or thighs, and feels at first like bad period pain. Any bleeding or spotting from the vagina in the first 28 weeks of pregnancy is called a threatened miscarriage.

Bleeding does not mean you are bound to lose the pregnancy. Many pregnant women, perhaps 50 per cent, have some bleeding and less than half of these will go on to miscarry. There are other possible causes of bleeding in pregnancy. It might be caused by a cervical erosion, a patch of red mucus-producing tissue on the cervix that may bleed spontaneously or when touched. It might be caused by a polyp, a non-cancerous growth that again may bleed readily. If you have cystitis, there may be bleeding which does not come from the vagina, but from the urethra. Even when the bleeding is coming from inside the uterus, miscarriage is not inevitable. Some women lose a great deal of blood and still go on to have healthy full-term babies.

What other signs of miscarriage are there? Many women describe feeling unwell for several days before a miscarriage. They may feel vaguely ill or sick or have flu-like symptoms. Or they may feel less sick as the symptoms of pregnancy fade. Or they may have an intuition that something is wrong. Sometimes the fear that something is wrong starts much earlier in the pregnancy. As Mary said, 'Deep down I just knew that once again it was a hopeless pregnancy.'

Yet healthy pregnancies have their share of unwell feelings and stomach pains. Feelings of foreboding are common too and many pregnant women fear at some time in the pregnancy that the baby has died. None of these feelings proves that a miscarriage is going to happen. And in at least half of all pregnancies that do threaten to miscarry, the bleeding stops and the woman goes on to give birth to a healthy baby.

No damage is done to the baby by a threatened miscarriage. The bleeding is caused by a small part of the placenta separating from the wall of the uterus, so the blood loss is from the mother, not the baby. If you had bled early in pregnancy, you have a slightly increased risk of having a premature labour or problems with placental function later in pregnancy, but there is no increased risk that the baby will be abnormal.

Bleeding after 28 weeks is called an ante-partum haemorrhage. What happens after 28 weeks is outside the scope of this book, but it is important to know that an ante-partum haemorrhage, unlike threatened miscarriage, may occasionally put the mother's life at risk. So if you have any bleeding after 28 weeks you should immediately contact your doctor or the obstetric unit at the hospital.

INEVITABLE MISCARRIAGE

If a woman is threatening to miscarry, there may come a point of no return. This is when the cervix starts to dilate. Once this action starts, there is no hope of saving the baby. For the miscarriage to take place, the cervix — the neck of the womb — has to be open to let the fetus through. The process involves both an opening up and a thinning out of the tissues of the cervix. Imagine putting on a tight polo-neck sweater — to allow your head through, the material must stretch and thin out as the neck opens up. As long as the cervix remains closed, the miscarriage is still only threatening to happen, but once the cervix starts to stretch out and open up, miscarriage is considered inevitable.

There are other signs too that you are probably going to miscarry. You may start to shiver and may feel or be sick. You may pass pieces of tissue, sometimes described as looking like raw liver. The pain may become more severe, as the uterus contracts to push out the contents just as in a full-term labour. The amount of pain varies considerably, from woman to woman, and from miscarriage to miscarriage. It can be severe and it is important that women be offered effective pain relief.

When a miscarriage threatens, often the main feeling is one of fear. Fear that you will lose the baby. Fear about the physical process of miscarriage, about the way your body seems to have taken over, against your will. Miscarriage is a process over which you have no control. There may also be a sense of shock and disbelief. Susan said, 'I remember saying to my husband "This is not me." I thought I would wake up in the morning at home.'

ADVICE

'Vaginal bleeding in pregnancy should always be taken seriously.' These words, or some variation on them, can be found in virtually every book or pamphlet aimed at pregnant women. For most of us, 'taking it seriously' means ringing the doctor. However, there is nothing a doctor can do to stop a miscarriage from happening and for this reason, many doctors do not admit women with early uncomplicated miscarriages to hospital. Some, rather than visiting, may give advice over the phone, at least at first. If your pregnancy is further advanced your doctor should see you to ascertain exactly what is happening as quickly as possible.

Most doctors will advise you to avoid sex until at least 48 hours after the bleeding has stopped. It is important to follow this advice, because if your cervix has started to dilate, you are at risk of infection.

Some doctors will also suggest you stay in bed, although others now question the usefulness of this advice. None of the doctors I consulted for the book felt that there was any value in bed-rest. Controversy between doctors means confusion for patients, and the woman who does lose her baby may wonder if she was given the wrong advice. As there seems to be no evidence that bed-rest could save a pregnancy, the best advice is to follow your own inclinations. You may choose to go to bed because you feel tired or ill, or because you feel safer there, but if you don't want to go to bed, there is no need to worry that you are increasing the risk of inevitable miscarriage.

MEDICAL RESPONSES

If you are showing signs of miscarrying, the doctor will try to find out what is happening by means of a variety of tests, depending on how far your pregnancy has advanced, and whether or not you are in hospital. You may be given an internal examination, a scan, a test to check for the baby's heartbeat or a pregnancy test. The doctor probably will not try to change the course of what is happening.

The internal examination will show whether or not the cervix is dilated. If the cervix is opening, a miscarriage is inevitable. There are two parts to the examination. For the first part, the doctor will use a speculum, a metal or plastic instrument with two arms that swing on a fulcrum. The speculum holds apart the walls of the vagina, enabling the doctor to see the cervix. He or she will also assess the size of the uterus by inserting the index and middle fingers of one hand into the vagina and placing the other hand on your lower abdomen, so that the uterus can be felt through the abdominal wall.

Some women worry that the internal examination can itself trigger miscarriage (see Chapter 5). Women may also complain that the examination is painful if they are in the process of miscarrying. The availability of ultrasound has made the internal examination less crucial in the diagnosis of miscarriage. If you are bleeding and would prefer not to have an internal examination, ask your doctor to postpone it and wait to see what happens.

Over the past few years, the ultrasound scan has become the obstetrician's main diagnostic tool. Ultrasound scanning works on the same principle by which submarines navigate and bats fly. Echoes of high frequency sound waves are used to build up a picture of what is happening inside the womb. If a scan is decided on at the hospital, you will be asked to drink a lot, as a full bladder pushes the womb up higher, so giving a clearer picture. Then you will be asked to lie flat on a couch, and your stomach will be gently oiled. Next a machine called a 'transducer' is passed over your abdomen, beaming ultrasonic sound waves, too high to hear, into your womb. The waves pass easily through fluid but bounce back off the solid surfaces of the fetus and the placenta, and the pattern of reflected sound is translated into a picture on a television screen. The picture is blurred, but a trained ultrasonographer will usually be able to tell whether there is a fetus, whether it is the right size, and whether it is alive as the heartbeat can be seen after about eight weeks of pregnancy.

However scans are not foolproof. The picture is not always clear and there may be difficulty in interpreting it. For this reason, action is never based on one picture.

Looking at the picture on the screen can be very distressing, as Tina's story shows. Tina had been bleeding and had been kept in hospital. One morning, the baby's heartbeat could not be found.

My specialist arrived with a portable ultrasound scanner and, with words of comfort, proceeded. In hope and despair I forced myself to look at the screen. Where there had been lively movement of arms and legs there was none — no movement at all, his little body was deathly still. Frantically I searched for a little sign, just something to say all was not lost. ... I had two more scans that day to make quite sure medically, these times I couldn't look, I needed no confirmation, the picture was vividly etched on my mind, a stillness never to be forgotten.

Another machine that may be used, particularly if the hospital or clinic does not have a scanner, is a Sonicaid fetal heart detector. This is a portable electronic device which is placed on the woman's stomach, and which picks up and amplifies the baby's heartbeat.

A pregnancy test may be done in the same circumstances as a scan — that is, if a missed miscarriage is suspected, or if a woman has had a threatened miscarriage and it is not clear whether or not the fetus has been expelled. The laboratory test, like the test you can do at home, measures human chorionic gonodatrophin (HCG), a hormone found in the urine of pregnant women. Like the scan, pregnancy testing is not totally reliable. It is possible to get a false positive reading for several days after miscarriage or after the death of a baby in the womb, as it takes some days for HCG to be cleared from the body. So several tests may be done on successive days.

All these tests can be very harrowing — despair is replaced by guarded hope, then yet another result brings your hopes crashing down again — but the care over the results is crucial. If a D & C or induction of labour is being considered, one question will preoccupy you: How can I be really sure that the baby is dead? The use of different kinds of tests, and repetitions of those tests, means that in the end there can be no doubt what has happened.

WHAT IS LOST DURING MISCARRIAGE?

It is natural to feel fear about what will come out during a miscarriage. The insides of our bodies are mysterious to us, inspiring a mixture of fascination and repulsion. In particular, the beginnings of new life inside women's bodies inspire a deep awe and fear. Many women know that miscarriages often happen because something is wrong with the baby, and fear that they will be confronted with something distorted, ugly, horribly malformed if they miscarry.

The most obvious loss from a miscarriage is blood. There may seem to be a great deal of it, as it is mixed up with amniotic fluid, the liquid that surrounds the fetus in its sac. The blood may be brownish or bright red. It usually becomes bright red later in the miscarriage, if not at the start. The blood may contain clots which are pieces of tissue. Often you will not see the form of the fetus at all. Sometimes there is not a fetus to see. Perhaps the fertilized egg scarcely developed at all, or perhaps the fetus died in early pregnancy and has dissolved away. In these cases a woman will just see blood with some clots or lumps of tissue.

Sometimes — especially with late miscarriages — women do see their babies. Here are some of their descriptions:

Tiny but complete and incredibly beautiful.

So beautiful and absolutely perfect, down to her tiny toenails.

It wasn't at all what I expected, it was so round and perfect and I was very proud of it and admired what we'd achieved.

He's got his eyes, his fingernails, fingers and a little stump of his sex organ and a little white cord ... All I wanted to do was to tell my husband and friends how lovely he was.

Seeing the baby may be shocking at the time, yet it seems to be an experience which women never regret. It is easier to grieve for a baby you see, however tiny. There is comfort, too, in knowing that your baby did not look deformed or ugly. Like the women quoted here, women often remark on how beautiful their baby was, and how perfectly formed.

Advice given to women who have miscarried may include the instruction that the fetus and any tissue or clots passed should be kept and taken to the doctor. The theory behind this advice is that the fetus can be tested for genetic defects. Perhaps 50 per cent of first trimester miscarriages are caused by such defects in the fetus. What the test cannot tell you is where the defect came from. Usually these defects are 'random' events, but occasionally they are caused by a problem in one of the parents' chromosomes. If such a problem is the reason for the miscarriage, then the same thing could happen again and the parents will need genetic counselling. However it is impossible to tell from the fetus alone whether or not one of the parents has such a problem. In order to be sure, the parents themselves have to be tested. So the woman who is unable to or chooses not to keep any tissue she miscarries has no need to worry that an important chance has been missed. And women who do take care to keep any tissue they pass may be disappointed in the results of the tests, as Caroline recalls: 'We took the baby with us to the hospital. I was desperate to know as much as possible about what might be wrong. The consultant said it was best not to try to understand these things — meaning miscarriages — as it was just a psychological prop. He said that the baby appeared to be perfectly normal and that he could give no explanation as to why it happened.'

When a woman miscarries before 28 weeks of pregnancy, there is no legal requirement about what should happen to the baby's remains. If a woman miscarries in hospital, any tissue that she miscarries that is not taken to be tested will be put in the hospital incinerator. It can be very distressing to think of your baby's remains being disposed of without ceremony. Women sometimes worry about what happens to the ashes, but there will be no ashes, as the tiny fetus has no bone. Women may also worry that the fetus might be stored on a laboratory shelf and used for teaching or research, but this would be very rare. If you are worried about this, it might help to raise your concerns with a sympathetic doctor.

Once the baby's body is taken by the hospital, it belongs to them. The assumption is that the woman has given it to the hospital and she cannot ask for it back later. However women do have the right to take the baby to bury themselves, if they decide that is what they want to do at the time of the miscarriage. Medical staff are unlikely to tell you that you have this alternative, and the woman who is numb and shocked after miscarriage is scarcely likely to ask.

Janet was one woman who did ask:

> There was one night sister who heard that I wanted to bury the baby. She asked me where, and I said 'the garden' as I had no idea where else. She said it was illegal to bury human tissue in the garden. I was adamant that I wanted to bury the baby, so said we'd contact the local cemetery. She said I must have confirmation that it was possible to bury a 15-week-old baby by midday that day. This was at 3.00 am and I had just miscarried. .... All the other nurses were reassuring that I could bury the baby, but didn't know what the procedure to release the baby from the hospital was. Luckily a woman doctor on the ward was sympathetic, and managed to get through the red tape, after my partner got a letter from the cemetery saying we had bought a space in a public grave for the baby.

For one woman, what happens to the fetus will be very important. For another, the 'products of conception' will have little significance once she knows that the baby is lost to her. We differ in the meanings we attach to these things. It is perhaps comparable with how we feel after a close relative or friend has died. For one person, it is important to see the body, and the ceremony associated with the body matters, while for another, the body has little significance once life has gone. There is no right reaction, but it is important at least to know the choices available to us.

TREATMENT AFTER MISCARRIAGE

Miscarriage does no harm to the mother's body. It does not in any way affect her chances of getting pregnant again and, generally, it does not take her very long to recover physically.

However there are two possible complications after miscarriage — severe bleeding and infection. These problems may arise if the uterus does not expel everything completely and fragments of the fetus or placenta are left inside. This situation is called an 'incomplete miscarriage'.

The fetus and placenta are fed by blood vessels. When they start to break up in the course of miscarriage there will be bleeding from open blood vessels and this will continue while bits of tissue remain in the uterus. During this time, too, the uterus is vulnerable to infection, rather like a bleeding cut before it scabs over.

Because of the risk of severe bleeding and infection, a D & C (or 'scrape') will always be done if there is any danger that fragments of tissue are left inside the uterus, or if the uterus has failed to expel the fetus (in other words, if there has been a missed or incomplete miscarriage). D & C stands for Dilatation and Curettage. It involves stretching the cervix ('dilatation') and scraping the inner lining of the uterus ('curettage'). The opening in the cervix is normally tiny, just wide enough to allow menstrual fluid through, but the opening can be gently stretched to allow a curette, an instrument rather like a long spoon, through to clean out the uterus.

Doctors disagree about whether a D & C is always necessary. If the cervix is closed — back to its normal diameter — it is very unlikely that there is any tissue still inside. This is a 'complete miscarriage'. An internal examination by a doctor will reveal if the cervical canal is closed. However some doctors believe that no miscarriage is complete until a D & C has been performed, as there is always a risk of tissue being left inside.

If a D & C is decided on, it is a very quick and simple operation, normally done under a light general anaesthetic. The woman is asked not to eat or drink anything for six hours before the operation because of the anaesthetic. The whole operation only takes a few minutes and the woman will usually be able to go home the day after the operation.

In the case of a 'missed miscarriage', the uterus will always have to be emptied, usually by means of a D & C. However if the pregnancy had progressed up to or beyond about week 16 before miscarrying labour will have to be induced. Prostaglandin hormone is administered either via a small tube (catheter) passed through the cervix, or via an intravenous drip. Another hormone, oxytocin, which makes the womb contract, may also be used together with the prostaglandin.

In cases of missed miscarriage, some doctors decide not to act immediately, preferring to wait and see whether 'nature takes its course' and the woman's body expels the fetus without any medical interference. For the woman involved, this is an extremely distressing situation. A woman who knows she is carrying a dead baby inside her will be desperate to have the situation brought to an end. Women with missed miscarriages sometimes have great difficulty in impressing their needs on the medical staff. Thelma had to face this problem:

> The last scan showed that my body had shed part of the embryo but not all. I was told I would need a D & C and was given an appointment for three weeks later by the out-patients' receptionist. I screamed at her, 'I can't walk around like this for three weeks!' My husband made arrangements for a D & C just one week later. During that time I would neither see nor speak to anyone but my husband. I felt 'taboo'. I had part of a dead person inside me.

Another possible treatment after miscarriage is the anti-D injection, given to the 15 per cent of women whose blood is rhesus negative. This measure is necessary to safeguard future pregnancies. Blood cells from the baby in the uterus can pass into the woman's bloodstream when the placenta breaks away during miscarriage. If the woman's blood is rhesus negative and the baby's blood is rhesus positive, the woman will develop antibodies to the rhesus-positive blood cells. Once these antibodies are in her blood stream they will remain there, and they will attack the red blood cells of any rhesus-positive baby she carries in the future. Any future babies she has might become anaemic in the womb and would require urgent treatment at birth. Treatment with anti-D gamma globulin destroys any rhesus-positive red blood cells that may have entered her blood stream during the miscarriage. The injection will also have to be given after any further miscarriages she has, or if she gives birth to a rhesus-positive child.

To be on the safe side, the anti-D injection should be given to any rhesus-negative woman who might have had a miscarriage — however early — even if it is not certain that she was in fact pregnant.[2] If you are rhesus negative, or don't know your blood group, you should see your doctor immediately if you think you may have miscarried. The injection must be given within 72 hours of the miscarriage.

PRODUCING MILK

The later your miscarriage, the more likely it becomes that you will produce milk. Of women who miscarry at 12 weeks, only about one in ten will produce milk, but it happens to the majority of women who miscarry at 19 weeks. If milk is going to come in, it will happen between two and five days after the miscarriage.

The sensation of milk coming in varies from mild discomfort to pain. There may be a tight or hot feeling in your breasts, and possibly some swelling. It is important to resist the urge to express (squeeze out) the milk, as you will only produce more. Some women have found it helpful to wear a tight, firm bra, and to shower their breasts with cold water. You may also need to take a painkiller such as Paracetomol. After a few days, your body should adjust and stop producing milk.

Having your breasts swell up with milk when you have lost your baby will be emotionally as well as physically painful. Your milk is flowing freely, yet there is no baby to feed.

SEX

Women are usually advised to avoid sexual intercourse until the bleeding stops, because of the risk of infection. There is no risk in forms of sexual activity that do not involve vaginal penetration.

Later I will discuss the reasons why it is a good idea to leave a gap before getting pregnant again. If you are going to follow this advice and use contraception, it is important to start straight after a miscarriage, as you can ovulate at any time. If you use a diaphragm or cervical cap, you should have the size checked after a miscarriage. If you are on the pill, you can start taking it the day after a miscarriage, but you should use some other form of contraception as well for a month. If you are going to use a coil or IUD you should wait for six weeks after miscarriage before having it fitted, as your uterus will still be soft and there is a slightly increased risk of perforation when the IUD is put in. In the meantime, you should use some other form of contraception.

AFTER-EFFECTS OF A MISCARRIAGE OR D & C

Bleeding after a miscarriage or D & C normally stops completely after two to three weeks, or even sooner. During this time, you should use sanitary towels, not tampons. If you had a D & C, you may feel tired and sleepy for several days because of the general anaesthetic.

After a miscarriage, you should contact your doctor if the bleeding goes on for longer than two to three weeks, is heavier than a normal menstrual flow, has clots in it or is very smelly. Any of these signs may indicate that there are still fragments of tissue left in your uterus, and you may need another D & C. You should also contact your doctor if you develop a temperature, or are experiencing pain that is worse than mild discomfort, or you simply do not feel well and cannot explain why. It may mean you have an infection and need treatment with antibiotics.

See your doctor immediately if you are worried.

TAKING TIME OFF WORK

After a miscarriage, your doctor may not suggest taking some time off work. Grace asked her doctor how long it should be before she went back to work and received the answer 'First thing Monday morning — after all, you have only lost a baby, nothing serious . . .'

The physical after-effects of miscarriage are usually short-lived, and you can go back to work just as soon as you feel physically ready. However, even if you feel quite energetic and positive, it is wise to take some time off work. You have been through an experience which most women find very distressing. Taking sick leave is a way of acknowledging the significance of what has happened. If your doctor does not offer sick leave, ask for it. Take yourself seriously and give yourself time to begin to recover.

FEELINGS

Crying, grieving, shock, not being able to believe it has happened — women describe all these reactions immediately after miscarriage. For some women, there may also be a more surprising feeling — a sense of relief. The physical stress and pain of the miscarriage are over. After everything you have been through you are still alive. Life goes on and still holds possibilities for you.

Sarah had her miscarriage induced at five months after two

days of intermittent contractions and bleeding. She had a 'short but incredibly painful labour. But oh! the relief when it was all over! My intravenous drip was removed, the contractions had ceased, and I could actually move around freely without feeling any pain! For the rest of that day and the duration of the next, the relief of pain counteracted any other negative emotions: I suppose I was in a kind of shock.' It was only several days later that Sarah started to grieve.

I remember those feelings of relief from my own miscarriages. I remember a feeling, too, about my body — how flat, empty, ordinary it felt. Almost as though the pregnancy had never happened. This is how Pamela McDonald put it:[3]

> They let me go home the next morning. I started to dress in the clothes I had worn to the hospital and for the first time I realized that my small bump wasn't there and there wasn't anything to carry out with me either, no small bundle wrapped in a blanket, just myself and my empty arms.

SOURCES

H.J. Huisjes, *Spontaneous Abortion*, Churchill Livingstone, Edinburgh, 1984

Gillian C.L. Lachelin, *Miscarriage, The Facts*, Oxford University Press, 1985

Ann Oakley, Ann McPherson and Helen Roberts, *Miscarriage*, Fontana, Glasgow, 1984

Hank Pizer and Christine O'Brien Palinski, *Coping with a Miscarriage*, Jill Norman, London, 1980

REFERENCES

1. Statistics quoted in Lachelin, *op cit*
2. Huisjes, *op cit*, p. 159
3. Pamela McDonald, 'Diary of a miscarriage', *Irish Times*, September 1981

2.
NORMAL PREGNANCY

... velvet footed, musing of my own,
Torpid, mellow, stupid as a stone.
GENEVIEVE TAGGARD, *With Child*

When I went home after my first miscarriage, my mind was full
of questions. What caused it? Was it something I had done?
Why did it happen to me? Will it happen again?

After a miscarriage, women are hungry for answers to
questions like these. Yet most of us will never find precise
answers. Some women do, but they are the exceptions, the ones
with the more unusual problems. Most of us will never know
exactly what caused our miscarriages. Even if I had been given
a whole battery of medical tests after my first miscarriage, it is
unlikely that I would have been given a satisfactory
explanation.

Even if we cannot get the kind of personal information we
would like, there is another kind of information that may be
helpful. Our hunger for knowledge can be at least partially
satisfied by finding answers to more general questions. What is
known about the possible causes of miscarriage? What are the
chances of it happening again for women with my kind of
history? Is there anything I can do to improve my chances next
time?

Women sometimes feel almost ashamed about their
desperate need for information after miscarriage, and the
lengths to which they will go to get it — spending hours in
bookshops, going to medical libraries and hunting through
medical textbooks, squandering money on expensive magazines
because the word 'miscarriage' appears on the cover. Yet it
makes complete sense that we should crave information as we
do. Finding answers at least to some of your questions helps you
cope. Knowledge helps you to deal with some of the painful
emotional after-effects of miscarriage — the guilt about the past

and the worry about the future. The more you know, the less likely you are to blame yourself for what has happened. And the more you know, the less likely you are to be plagued by unnecessary fears in your next pregnancy. You will still worry, of course, but you will at least have the confidence that comes from knowing what you can do something about, and what is outside your control.

To understand the possible causes of miscarriage, it is essential to have some background information. We need to know about normal pregnancy, before we can understand what happens when something goes wrong.

When I had my first miscarriage, I had very little idea what went on inside my body to produce a period or a pregnancy. My knowledge was limited to dimly remembered diagrams in school biology books, and I found it very hard to relate those vague images to my own body. Most of the organs concerned are hidden and inaccessible. I could not imagine what they looked like, or what size they were, or quite how they were connected up. I had still less idea precisely how they worked, or what part they played in menstruation, pregnancy or miscarriage.

I don't think I was unusual. Women generally know surprisingly little about their bodies. I imagine our lack of knowledge has its roots in attitudes to women's bodies, in our own culture and probably in most other cultures too. As girls we learn very quickly that the workings of female bodies are a source of embarrassment and must be hidden or ignored. Little girls are discouraged from exploring themselves. Periods and 'women's troubles' are talked about in hushed voices, or not at all. We feel uncomfortable about touching our genitals, and our first efforts at putting in a tampon or using a diaphragm or cap are often fumbling, nervous and unsuccessful. Our ignorance about how our bodies work is perhaps all part of this embarrassment and shame about our sexual and reproductive organs. It is as though the 'Keep Off' command applies not just to our hands, but to our minds as well.

Hopefully this chapter will fill in some of the gaps and supply that essential background information.

THE FEMALE REPRODUCTIVE ORGANS

The female organs involved in conception and pregnancy are the ovaries, Fallopian tubes, uterus, cervix and vagina.

The ovaries are situated a few inches below the woman's waist, and are about 3-4 cm (1.5 in) long and the shape of almonds. They act as the storehouses for the eggs or ova, which were made in the first weeks of a woman's own life in the womb.

These immature ova, together with their packaging of smaller cells are called follicles. When a baby girl is born, she already has about 400,000 ova in her ovaries, but only about 400 will develop into mature ova. An ovum is a single cell. Cells, which are the basic unit of all living things, are very tiny — most are so small that they can only be seen under the microscope — but a mature ovum is as large as a full stop on this page.

The Fallopian tubes are about 10 cm (4 in) long and it is in one of these that fertilization takes place. One end of the tube is next to but not actually connected to the ovary, and fringed to catch the mature ovum released by the ovary. The tube narrows towards the uterus and the opening to the uterus is so tiny that only a very fine needle could pass through it.

In a woman who is not pregnant, the uterus or womb is about the size and shape of a pear. Its walls are muscular — in fact the uterus is one of the most powerful muscles in the body, capable of the tremendous force of movement that is required to push a baby out. The walls of the uterus have a soft velvety lining of spongy tissue called the endometrium. The muscle walls and the spongy lining are connected by a dense network of tiny blood vessels.

The cervix is the neck of the uterus. If you have ever used a diaphragm, you will have learned to find the cervix with your finger. It feels like a round knob with a dimple in its centre. This dimple is the os, the tiny opening that connects the inside of the uterus with the vagina.

The vagina is about 7.5-10 cm (3-4 in) long. It is lined with ribbed tissue and has very elastic walls. The vagina is constantly moistened by secretions that help keep it clean and help prevent infections. The vagina ends in the outer genitals, known as the vulva, consisting of the outer labia (or lips), the inner labia, and the clitoris which is the most sensitive spot and the primary source of sexual pleasure.

A woman's entire menstrual cycle is under the control of hormones. These are chemical messengers that are made in one part of the body and carried in the blood to affect the workings of organs in another part of the body. Some hormones are made by the ovaries, others by the pituitary gland in the brain.

A NORMAL MONTHLY CYCLE

In the first days of a woman's period or menstrual bleeding, a hormone is produced by her body which signals the start of the new cycle. This hormone is called follicle stimulating hormone (FSH) and its name describes exactly what it does. FSH acts on one of the ovaries, stimulating the growth of some of the

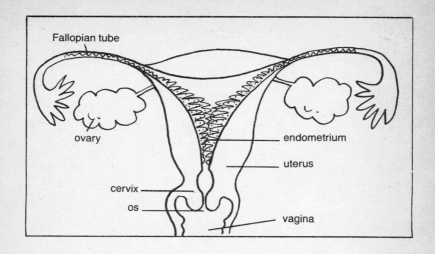

FIGURE 1 The female reproductive organs

follicles. A number of follicles start growing, but for reasons we do not know, one alone grows more rapidly than the others. As it matures this follicle moves towards the outer wall of the ovary. When another chemical signal comes, this time of luteinizing hormone (LH), the follicle breaks, releasing the mature ovum. This moment is ovulation.

The ovum floats out of the follicle, in the direction of the Fallopian tube. There is a gap between the ovary and the tube, but the tube has fringed ends that move like fingers to draw the ovum into the tube. Once safely inside the tube, the ovum is moved down towards the uterus by hairlike cells that line its walls and by wavelike movements of the tube.

Some women know when they are ovulating. They notice a different kind of vaginal discharge, a clear, slightly elastic mucus that looks like raw egg white. They may get some back pain or a little bleeding. The clearest signal of all that a woman has ovulated is a slight rise in her body temperature. One of the first suggestions a doctor will make if you are having difficulty in conceiving will be for you to take your temperature with a special fertility thermometer throughout the month, to find out whether and when you are ovulating.

The discarded follicle still has an important role to play. It is now called the corpus luteum, or 'yellow body', because it contains yellow fat. It produces the hormone progesterone, which is crucial in early pregnancy. If the ovum is not fertilized,

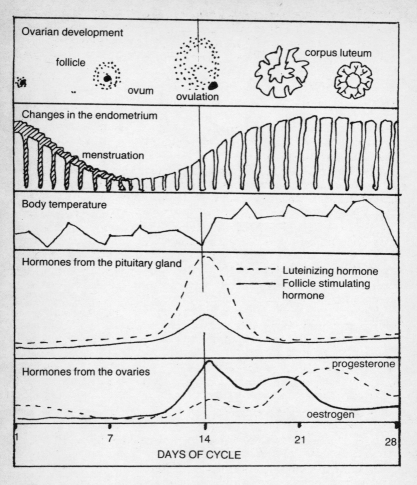

FIGURE 2 The normal menstrual cycle

production of progesterone peaks between ten and six days before the next period, then dies away, and the 'yellow body' disintegrates and disappears.

If the ovum does not meet with any sperm on the way, it travels on down the Fallopian tube and into the uterus. In response to hormonal signals the lining of the uterus has gradually thickened during the month, in readiness to receive a fertilized ovum. If the ovum has not been fertilized, this rich lining of blood cells is no longer required and will eventually be shed through the vagina as a normal period. The blood flow will wash out from the uterus whatever remains of the unfertilized egg. After a day or two of the menstrual flow, the hormonal changes cause a new follicle to start growing and the whole cycle begins again.

FERTILIZATION

What happens if a woman makes love at the right time? What if the ovum meets with sperm on the course of its journey down the Fallopian tube?

If the ovaries are storehouses, then the man's testes are factories, making millions of sperm from puberty virtually to the end of his life. Sperm are minute cells, much smaller than the ova. Where a mature ovum is as big as a full stop, a sperm is 100,000 times smaller than that. In a single ejaculation, there may be a mind-boggling 200 million of them.

For the ovum to be fertilized, the ovum and sperm must meet up in the Fallopian tube. This means the sperm have a long way to go. They have to make their way from the top of the vagina, where they are deposited during sexual intercourse, through the os (the opening in the cervix) into the uterus, then through the uterus and out into the Fallopian tube.

Of all the millions of sperm that go on this journey, very few make it to the Fallopian tube and only one actually penetrates the membrane that surrounds the egg. The long hard journey has been seen as a built-in safety mechanism. The picture is of a kind of endurance test or marathon race, with the feeble or sickly sperm being weeded out, and the strongest healthiest sperm winning the prize. It is an attractive idea, but there is no evidence for it. Unfortunately abnormal sperm do sometimes fertilize the ovum.[1]

So finally ovum and sperm unite. These two separate cells, which in some unknown way have been seeking each other out, come together to form a new life. The tiny translucent cell formed by their fusion is at the very start of an extraordinary process of growth. In the course of the pregnancy, that single cell will grow into a baby with two thousand million cells in his or her body.

THE GROWTH OF THE EMBRYO

The fertilized cell immediately divides up to form two cells. Ovum and sperm were completely different from one another, but these two new cells are identical. To picture how two identical cells can be made from two different ones, imagine taking a glass of water and a glass of ink, and mixing them together, and then dividing the mixture up again.

The process of dividing up continues in the Fallopian tube — first two cells, then four, then eight. After about four days, the embryo, as the baby is known for the first five weeks of its development, still consisting of only a small number of cells arrives at the uterus, where it has to make a home for itself until the moment of birth. The lining of the uterus, as we have seen, has been thickening in response to hormonal signals in this part of the woman's cycle. It has an enriched blood supply and glands that secrete all the nourishment the growing embryo will need. The process by which the embryo settles into the lining of the womb is called 'implantation', or 'embedding', or 'nidation' — which means nesting.

The lining of the uterus then grows over the embryo and fastens it securely. The connection between mother and baby is now in place for the duration of the pregnancy. So far all the cells have been identical, but at this point two different kinds of cells start to develop. Some form the organs of the embryo and some form the placenta that later in pregnancy will nourish and protect the baby.

MAINTAINING THE PREGNANCY

The womb provides one of our most basic images of safety and security. Phrases like 'back to the womb' suggest a state of total peace and harmony, and protection from all the troubles and trials of life in the world outside. However to maintain the embryo in the womb safely, a number of delicate and complex mechanisms — many of them still not fully understood — have to keep working in perfect balance.

Hormones have a crucial role to play in maintaining the pregnancy. Progesterone, in particular, is very important in early pregnancy. This is the hormone that causes the glands in the lining of the uterus to secrete their nutrients and ensures that the lining has a good blood supply. Progesterone has a tranquillizing effect and is probably responsible for the feeling of peacefulness that many women enjoy when pregnant. In very early pregnancy, progesterone is still being produced by the corpus luteum, the 'yellow body' that remains in the ovary in pregnancy instead of dying off as it does in the course of a normal menstrual cycle. Later, perhaps 10 or 12 weeks after the first day of a woman's last period, the placenta takes over the production of progesterone.

Another hormone produced in early pregnancy is HCG, human chorionic gonadotrophin. This causes the corpus luteum to persist and produce the crucial progesterone and oestrogen, necessary for the maintenance of the pregnancy. If you have ever used a home pregnancy test kit, you will have seen HCG in action. It is the HCG in a pregnant woman's urine that cause those thrilling or worrying changes in the test-tube.

Hormones are understood quite well, but there are other aspects of pregnancy that remain largely mysterious. One question that particularly perplexes scientists at the moment is why the bundle of cells is not immediately rejected when it is first formed. Our bodies are programmed to recognize and reject any foreign cells — for instance, viruses, bacteria, organs transplanted from somebody else's body. This defence mechanism is called the immune system. The fertilized ovum gets half its chromosomes from the father. From what is known of how the immune system works, the mother's body should instantly reject this half-foreign object, but in a normal pregnancy, there are subtle changes in the woman's immune system which include the production of substances which stop this process of rejection from taking place. However, as yet very little is known about these crucial substances and how they work, or why in some instances, they fail to work.

CHROMOSOMES

Chromosomes give a new cell its instructions for action. There are 46 of them in every cell in the body — except, as we shall see, for the ovum and the sperm — and they are organized in pairs. If you look at a cell under a powerful microscope, you can see the chromosomes. They are thin strands of material, looking rather like a handful of twisted streamers after a children's party.

Chromosomes are responsible for all the characteristics we inherit from our parents and grandparents. A newborn baby can make us marvel at the working of the chromosomes, when she puckers up her face and suddenly looks exactly like her great-grandfather. At moments like that, we are aware of the precision of genetic inheritance.

Each chromosome is made up of thousands of different units or genes. Chromosomes are often likened to strands of beads, not unlike the popper necklace that little girls used to wear, made up of plastic beads that pop together and snap apart. If each chromosome is a necklace, then the genes are the individual beads. Each unit or bead contains a concise coded message. One gene, for instance, might contain instructions about hair colour, another about height, another about blood group, and so on.

The one tiny cell that is formed by the fusion of ovum and sperm will have multiplied to make two thousand million cells by the end of the pregnancy. It does this by a process of division called mitosis. First each chromosome in the cell has to make a copy of itself. Each of those strands of popper beads doubles itself. The strands of beads then coil together in pairs. There are now 92 chromosomes in each cell, divided up into 46 pairs. The pairs of chromosomes separate into two sets, each set destined for a separate cell. The sets of chromosomes move to opposite sides of the cell, then they break away from one another. Now there are two cells where before there was only one.

Looked at under the microscope, mitosis is like a complicated formation dance, involving a great deal of dividing, moving around and joining up again. It is easy to imagine how, as with formation dancing, one very small mistake can lead to chaos, and the earlier the mistake, the more cells that are affected. One wrong move by the genes and whole lines of cells will be faulty, with no possibility of the fault being put right.

Chromosomes in the ovum and the sperm

The ovum and the sperm are produced by a process of division that involves halving, a process known as meiosis. In the case of the ovum, this happened a long time ago, when the woman was herself still a baby in the womb. In the case of the sperm, it is happening all the time, from puberty virtually to the end of a man's life.

In meiosis, the process of division begins just as in mitosis. The chromosomes, the strands of beads, in one cell each make a copy of themselves. The strands coil together in pairs, and the pairs separate into two sets and divide up to form two new cells. Then those two cells divide up again but this time they do not double before they divide. So the chromosomal material is halved. There are now four cells, each with half the number of chromosomes — 23 instead of 46. All other cells in the body have 46 chromosomes, so the sperm and the ovum both need to unite with another cell with 23 chromosomes to make a complete cell.

The Greek philosopher Plato described love as the process of finding your other half, the person who would complete you. It is a theme that has been echoed by poets and song writers down the centuries. As far as our relationships are concerned, this is a more or less appealing poetic fiction, but it is literally true of the tiniest building blocks in the sexual organs. Sperm and ovum need each other to be complete. They are made for one another.

THE BACKGROUND TO MISCARRIAGE

In the course of this complicated and still mysterious process at the very start of a new life, much can go wrong. Something may be wrong with the ovum or sperm to start with, because there has been a mistake in the process of division by which the ovum or sperm was formed. The bundle of cells may fail to implant or may implant in the wrong place. Something may go wrong as the embryo grows, during that complex process of division from one cell to two thousand million. The growing embryo or fetus may not get enough nutrients from the mother's bloodstream or from the placenta. Something may go wrong with the process that stops the mother's body rejecting this foreign body that is growing inside her.

These possible problems give us clues to some of the causes of miscarriage.

SOURCES

Angela Phillips and Jill Rakusen (eds) *Our Bodies, Ourselves*, Penguin, Harmondsworth, 1979

Hank Pizer and Christine O'Brien Palinski, *Coping with a Miscarriage*, Jill Norman, London, 1980

REFERENCES

1.   G.W. Salisbury, R.G. Hart and J.R. Lodge, 'The spermatazoan genome and fertility', *American Journal of Obstetrics and Gynaecology*, vol. 128, pp. 342-50, 1977

3.
POISONS AND OTHER HAZARDS

... she had never forgotten that, if you drink much from a
bottle marked 'poison', it is almost certain to disagree with
you, sooner or later.
LEWIS CARROLL, *Alice's Adventures In Wonderland*

When I went to see my GP for an explanation after my first
miscarriage, he said, 'There was probably something wrong with
the fetus.' When I asked what that meant, I was told, 'It
probably had some sort of chromosomal abnormality.'

Chromosomal abnormalities, according to some studies,
account for more than half of all miscarriages. Most
chromosomal abnormalities are incompatible with life. Down's
Syndrome (which used to be called mongolism) is one example
of a chromosomal abnormality. It is an exception in that some
Down's Syndrome babies do survive, though most — perhaps
nine out of ten — are miscarried.

Chromosomal abnormalities can be seen under the
microscope. There are other kinds of genetic disorders which
cannot be so readily identified. Just one of the thousands of
genes may be defective. Some genetic defects may lead to
miscarriage, but with others the babies may survive. Muscular
dystrophy is one example of a genetic defect. Babies with
muscular dystrophy do survive pregnancy and birth, but
tragically they die in childhood.

In some miscarriages, there may be no fetus at all. This
situation is called a 'blighted ovum'. The cluster of cells never
gets beyond a very basic stage of development and the amniotic
sac may be virtually empty. 'Blighted ovum' may be something
of a misnomer, as it is probably the sperm that is 'blighted'. It is

thought that the problem arises when a normal ovum is fertilized by an abnormal sperm. All blighted ova are miscarried.

When I was told that my miscarried baby had probably had one of these problems, I asked what might have caused it. I was told that this was a 'random' event, but what does 'random' mean here?

Reproduction is an enormously wasteful business. As we have seen, a woman has thousands of ova in her ovaries, and every ejaculation contains millions of sperm. It is in the nature of things that some of the ova and some of the sperm will, by chance, be imperfect. If an imperfect ovum or sperm happens to be involved in fertilization, a miscarriage or birth defect will result. We have, of course, no control over this kind of unlucky accident, and no way of predicting when such an accident might occur.

It is known, however, that there are certain situations in which there is an increased risk that problems will arise. Agents that create such situations are called teratogens — radiation and certain chemicals, drugs and viruses would be examples of teratogens. If we imagine again that complex dance of the chromosomes, a teratogen might have the effect of, for instance, speeding up the music, or turning off the lights. It produces a situation in which the dancers are more likely to end up in the wrong place.

However — as is apparent from the case of the 'blighted ovum' — it is not just the fertilized ovum that can be damaged. The woman's ova and the man's sperm are vulnerable to damage before ever they meet up. The risks are different for men and women. The adult woman's ova are quite well protected, but if they do get damaged, for instance, by massive doses of radiation used in the treatment of cancer, they cannot regenerate, but remain damaged for the rest of the woman's reproductive life. The man's sperms are less well protected and more vulnerable to damage, but because the man keeps making new sperm, the damage is not permanent. If the agent causing the damage is removed, he will probably recover his capacity to produce normal sperm.

It is not just before and during fertilization that things can go wrong. There are other kinds of defects that can arise later, as the fetus develops. Exposure to a teratogen later in pregnancy may prevent a particular stage of development from progressing normally.

Up to day 17 from conception, all the cells in the embryo develop in the same way. (At day 17 the woman is about four and a half weeks pregnant. 'Weeks of pregnancy' means the number of weeks since the start of a woman's last menstrual period, so four weeks of pregnancy will, on average, be about two weeks from conception.) Then at day 18 — just around the time you are wondering what has happened to your period — comes a critical moment in the baby's life. The cells start to specialize, developing along different lines, differentiating into all the millions of kinds of cells that go to make up the various components of the human body. This development follows an orderly sequence. The precise damage caused by a teratogen will depend on its timing and which part of the sequence it interrupts. The thalidomide tragedy gives a clear example. The thalidomide babies were perfectly normal at conception, but thalidomide taken during the first trimester of pregnancy, when their arms and legs were developing, interrupted the sequence of development, so these babies were born with very short limbs.

'Neural tube defects' are the most common sort of developmental problem. Between 20 and 30 days after fertilization (five or six weeks of pregnancy) is a crucial time for the development of the brain, spinal cord and spine. At this time there is a major re-organization of the cells in the embryo: a sheet of cells folds over to form the tube that will make the brain and spinal cord. In neural tube defects, something happens at this point of pregnancy to stop development proceeding normally. In very severe cases most of the brain fails to develop. This is called 'anencephaly'. Alternatively the spine may fail to develop properly, as in cases of spina bifida. Most babies with neural tube defects are miscarried. At least one in ten miscarried fetuses have neural tube defects, and among poorly nourished women the proportion is much higher. In Northern Ireland, where spina bifida is common, one in three miscarried babies have neural tube defects.[1]

By day 55 from conception (about 10 weeks of pregnancy), the organs are mostly formed. The fetus is still sensitive to damage, but much less so than earlier in the pregnancy. Exposure to a teratogen at this stage might slow down the growth of the fetus, or damage its immature nervous system.

What do we know about teratogens? The information available can make depressing reading. The womb used to be thought of as a safe place. It was believed that the baby was protected from harm by the placental barrier, which filtered out any poisons or other harmful substances. Now, especially since the thalidomide tragedy, we know better. It is easy to despair. The baby in your womb may seem so vulnerable, and you may feel there is so little you can do to protect it. None of us can totally avoid exposure to some of these hazards, but do remember that, although severe exposure to a teratogen will to some extent increase the risk to your baby, it does not make damage inevitable.

TOXIC HAZARDS AT WORK

There is nothing new about toxic hazards in the workplace. Lewis Carroll's Mad Hatter demonstrated the effects of just such a toxic hazard. Hatters in Victorian times used a great deal of mercury in their work and many developed unpleasant symptoms, including mental disorders, as a result. And there is nothing new about the idea that toxins in the workplace might have an adverse effect on human reproduction. A hundred years ago, for instance, it was discovered that the children of male pottery workers exposed to lead had more birth defects than would be expected, and a death rate of one in two. When the mothers were exposed to lead, the effects were even more serious.

However what is new, over the past few decades, is the sheer variety of chemicals in use. There are now estimated to be 500,000 of them — and the number is growing all the time. Many of these substances have not been thoroughly tested for reproductive effects. And even where tests have been done, their validity may be in doubt — a major US chemical testing house, Industrial Bio-Test, was closed down after it was convicted of producing fraudulent results.

Even where hazards are recognized or suspected, workers cannot always rely on employers to protect them. In 1977, a group of men at an American plant making a pesticide — DBCP — started to talk to one another about their difficulty in having children. When their shop steward arranged for the workers to be tested, half of them were found to be sterile. Studies performed by the manufacturers in the 1950s had indicated that DBCP had a toxic effect on the testicles, but these findings were suppressed.[2] In 1977 manufacture of DBCP was stopped in the US, but the chemical plant was exported to a Third World country where restrictions are less stringent.

The story of DBCP makes it clear that it is not only women who are at risk from poisons at work. In other words, it is no solution to the problem just to protect women. Pregnant women are protected by law from excessive exposure to lead and radiation, and there have been suggestions that the problem of toxic hazards could be dealt with by banning pregnant women from working with other substances too. Yet this is no real solution. The man's sperm are just as vulnerable as the fetus. The fetus itself is most vulnerable right at the beginning of its life in the womb, before the woman even knows she is pregnant.

The only solution to the problem of toxic hazards is to make the workplace safe for *all* workers.

Here is a list of chemical substances which may have reproductive effects. New substances are coming into use all the time, so the absence of a name from the list does not mean it is safe. With some of these substances, there is only limited evidence of risk, but there is a good case for extra care in handling all of them.

Chemical substances for which there is some evidence of reproductive hazards

From 'Your reproductive health at risk' published by the General Municipal, Boilermakers' and Allied Trades Union

Acrylonitrile
Aniline
Anaesthetic Gases
Arsenic & compounds
 (e.g. sodium arsenate
 & arsenite)

Benzene
Benzo (a) pyrene
Beryllium
Boron (Boric Acid)

Cadmium
Carbon Disulphide
Carbon Monoxide
Chlordecone (Kepone)
Chloro-difluoromethane
Chloroform
Chloroprene

D.D.T.
Dibromochloropropane
Dichloromethane

Epichlorohydrin
Ethylene Dibromide
Ethylene Dichloride
Ethylene Oxide

Formaldehyde

Hexachloro-benzene

Lead (Inorganic &
 organic
Manganese
Mercury (organic &
 inorganic)
Methyle ethyl ketone
Monomethylformamide

Nitrogen Dioxide

Ozone

Polybrominated Biphenyls
 (PBB's)
Polychlorinated Biphenyls
 (PCB's)
Perchloroethylene
 (tetrachloroethylene)

Selenium and compounds

Tellurium
Thallium
Toluene

Vinyl Chloride
Warfarin

Xylene

What should you do if you suspect that you or your partner is
working with one of these substances, or with other suspect
chemicals?

It is important to find out all you can. Your employer should
tell you if you are working with any toxic chemical (Section 2(2)
of the Health and Safety at Work Act 1974). Suppliers or
manufacturers of chemicals used at work have to research into
the effects of their products. Your employers should therefore
have 'data sheets' on any chemical substances they buy to use
at work. If you are in a union, you have a right to appoint a
Safety Representative to take up issues like this. There may
well be one already at your place of work. Safety representatives
can ask the employer to see if anything used in the work context
may be a reproductive hazard. They can then negotiate with the
employer either for the removal of the hazard, or for better
safety precautions. Their best weapon in negotiating is the
Congenital Disabilities Act. Under this act, the employer can be
sued and made to pay heavy compensation if an employee's
baby is born with a handicap which can be traced to the
workplace.

Whatever kind of toxic hazard you are working with, once
you are pregnant, you have the right to be moved to a safer job
under the terms of the Employment Protection Act which
prevents your employer from sacking you because of your
pregnancy.

X-RAYS

Radiation is the transmission of any form of energy across space
without using wires or other physical carriers. There are two
basic kinds of radiation: ionizing radiation is a high frequency
form of energy, and includes nuclear radiation, X-rays and
ultra-violet light; non-ionizing radiation is of lower frequency,
and includes visible light, infra-red waves, microwaves and
radio waves.

The damage that ionizing radiation can cause to the baby in
the womb is well recognized. Ionizing radiation causes changes
in the structure of cells and a baby who is exposed to this kind
of radiation when in the womb has an increased risk of

developing childhood leukaemia. Animal experiments suggest that exposure to ionizing radiation in the womb causes a rise in numbers of miscarriages and birth defects. And ionizing radiation may also have mutagenic effects, in other words it causes changes in the structure of the genes which can be passed on down the generations.

Legislation and medical practice go some way to protect pregnant women from these effects. If a woman of child-bearing age needs a medical X-ray, it will be done during the first 10 days of her cycle, before she has ovulated. Permissible exposure levels for people exposed to X-rays in the course of their work, eg baggage handlers at airports, are especially low for pregnant women.

If you have had a number of X-rays in the past, there is no need to worry that this will increase your risk of miscarriage. Women who had repeated hip X-rays in childhood are no more likely to miscarry than other women.

VDUS

The last few years have seen the sudden development of new forms of office technology, with the result that few offices are now without VDUs. Since 1981, concern has grown that it is risky for pregnant women to work at or near VDUs. Many clusters of miscarriages, stillbirths and birth defects associated with VDUs have come to light. Here are a few: at a bank in Grimsby, between 1977 and 1978, of five women who became pregnant, three had miscarriages, one a stillbirth and one a deformed baby; at a Department of Employment in Runcorn, 20 out of 55 pregnancies between 1974 and 1982 resulted in miscarriage, stillbirth and/or malformation; in a survey of VDU users in the US, out of 800 women, 240 had had miscarriages and 54 had had babies with major birth deformities; at the Solicitor General's Office in Ottawa, Canada, seven out of eight pregnancies during 1979 and 1982 ended abnormally. All seven women involved worked on VDUs. The eighth gave birth to a healthy baby and did not work on a VDU. Statistically, the chances of some of the reported clusters being random occurrences are as low as six in a million.

Government and employers have so far failed to respond to women's well-founded anxieties. There are of course huge vested interests. Employers have invested millions of pounds in equipping their workplaces with computers and the futures of several multi-million pound electronic firms are dependent on them. The government sees the new technology as the foundation for our economic revival. So in spite of all the worrying evidence, the debate continues about the significance of these findings.

There has been a lot of discussion about safety levels. Attention has largely been focused on the ionizing radiation VDUs emit, and it has been argued that the levels are too low to cause harm. This may well be true, but VDUs also emit a number of other kinds of radiation, for instance, radio frequency (RF), very low frequency (VLF) and extremely low frequency (ELF), all of which have been shown to have some reproductive effects. In Czechoslovakia, women of child-bearing age are prohibited from working with RF radiation because of reports of increased numbers of miscarriages and birth defects. In Sweden a study established that children born to men who are exposed to ELF radiation in the course of their work have an increased incidence of congenital malformations.

One potentially damaging feature of the radiation emitted by VDUs is that it is 'pulsed', meaning that the energy is given off in short bursts. In a recent Swedish study, pregnant mice were exposed during the first 14 days of pregnancy to the kinds of pulsed radiation emitted by VDUs. The incidence of fetal malformations among the irradiated mice was four to five times higher than in a control group.[3]

Another possible hazard of VDUs has also been identified. Polychlorinated biphenyls (PCBs) are used in some VDUs as insulating fluids, and these chemicals can cause reproductive damage.

By and large it is women who work at VDUs for long periods of time, but the Swedish study is a reminder that men of course are not immune from the reproductive effects of radiation. One study found there were more birth defects among the offspring of male VDU operators than among those of women VDU operators.

The VDU Workers' Rights Campaign, set up in 1985, is demanding legislation to give pregnant women and those attempting to become pregnant the right to transfer to alternative work. They are also recommending that safer technology be developed, for instance liquid crystal display.

The VDU Workers' Rights Campaign offers this advice to pregnant women and those attempting to become pregnant:

1. Avoid unnecessary exposure to VDUs. Take coffee and lunch breaks away from the machine.
2. If possible, switch off the VDU when it is not in use.
3. Report any unusual medical symptoms to your health and safety officer and/or doctor.

4.   Ask your employer for details of the equipment's specification — is the flyback transformer shielded?

5.   Try to assess whether a VDU is really necessary for the job. Would an electronic memory typewriter do just as well?

6.   Try to find out from your employer if the VDU contains PCBs.
     It is well worth considering joining a union and reaping the benefits of collective bargaining.

If you work at a VDU, you could contact the VDU Workers' Rights Campaign for further information (see Useful Addresses).

ALCOHOL

One of the earliest warnings of the dangers of drinking alcohol around conception and during pregnancy can be found in the Old Testament. Samson's mother is told, 'Behold thou shalt conceive and bear a son, and now drink no wine or strong drink. ...' The risks were also recognized in Ancient Carthage where bridal couples were forbidden by law to drink on their wedding night, in case a handicapped child was conceived.

These old warnings have been heard again over the past few years. Since the 1970s, a number of studies have documented the damage that alcohol can do to the fetus. Alcohol is now recognized as a potential teratogen — a substance that can harm the baby in the womb.

Mothers who drink very heavily may give birth to babies suffering from Fetal Alcohol Syndrome. These babies have a range of problems, including reduced growth, damaged nervous systems and reduced intelligence. This syndrome is rare, but recently researchers have suggested that even social drinking may endanger the baby. One study concluded that the risk of miscarriage in the second trimester is doubled for women drinking one to two drinks daily, compared with non-drinkers.[4] (In this study, as in all research on the subject, one drink means ½ pint of beer, one glass of wine, one measure of spirits, or an equivalent amount of other forms of alcohol.) Another study found that even drinking just one or two drinks twice a week doubles the risk of miscarriage throughout pregnancy.[5]

Experts disagree on what advice should be given to women. The Royal College of Psychiatrists recommend pregnant women should be told not to drink at all, while the Royal College of Obstetrics and Gynaecology recommend that women should be advised to moderate their drinking in pregnancy. In practice, most GPs will recommend moderation rather than abstinence. Perhaps it is time for this advice to be changed. It is true that plenty of women who drink socially throughout pregnancy have healthy babies — alcohol, like other teratogens, affects different people in different ways — but the fact remains that the risks are considerable and women should be told about them. Many of us are more than willing to give things up while we are pregnant if we are given good reasons for it.

What about men? There have been few studies of the effects of male alcohol consumption on reproduction. Here we touch on a recurrent theme in this book: the failure of researchers to remember that men too play a part in reproduction. Yet it is known that men who drink heavily have more abnormal sperm, which may mean a higher risk of miscarriages and birth defects. Animal experiments back up the suggestion that heavy alcohol consumption in males may lead to miscarriage. When male mice were given alcohol before mating, there was an increased risk that some of the offspring of these mice would die in the mother's womb.[6] This result hints that some miscarriages may be caused by heavy drinking by the man during the three months before conception, when the sperm are being formed.

SMOKING

The first writer to suggest that tobacco may harm the fetus gives as his evidence an increase in the miscarriage rate. In his *Manual of Antenatal Pathology and Hygiene*, 1904, Ballantyne reported that women working in tobacco factories were more likely than other women to miscarry.

The risks of smoking in pregnancy are today well-known. Women who smoke often try to give up during pregnancy, and feel very guilty if they fail. The main known danger of smoking in pregnancy is that it may lead to a low birth-weight baby. Small babies are less robust than others, more at risk from infection, and more likely to die in the first few weeks of life. However smoking also produces an increased risk of miscarriage. One study found that women who smoked in pregnancy were almost twice as likely to have miscarriages as non-smoking women.[7]

Smoking causes cancer and any carcinogen could in theory cause genetic damage because of its effect on growing cells. So does smoking put up your risk of conceiving a baby with chromosomal abnormalities? The answer may be yes, when it is the man who smokes. One study found that men who smoked had a significantly higher proportion of abnormal sperm than men who did not.[8] But the answer is almost certainly no for women who smoke. Research suggests that women who smoke are no more likely than other women to have babies with chromosomal abnormalities. But they *are* more likely to miscarry normal fetuses.

If the damage is not chromosomal, what then is causing these miscarriages? One possibility is that the baby is being starved of oxygen and other nutrients while the mother smokes, as the carbon monoxide and nicotine in cigarette smoke may restrict blood flow and limit the blood's capacity to carry oxygen. As a result the baby does not grow as it should — it may even die. This theory would explain both the increased risk of miscarriage for women who smoke and the reduced birth weights of babies who are carried to term.

DISEASES

There would seem to be good reason for thinking that illness in the mother could cause miscarriage. One of the best known teratogens is a viral disease — rubella (German measles). Also, there are certain diseases known to cause miscarriage in animals, eg brucella abortus, so called because it causes miscarriage in cattle. And if you are feeling ill yourself, you are bound to worry that your illness will harm your baby. Occasionally your fears may be justified. Certain viruses can infect the baby and may lead to miscarriage, but fortunately this seems to be a rare occurrence. By and large the fetus seems to be well protected from the effects of the mother's illness.

Three viruses are known to cause congenital abnormalities and therefore may lead to increased risk of miscarriage. These are genital herpes, cytomegalovirus and rubella. You can protect yourself against rubella by having your immunity checked before becoming pregnant. If you had the injection more than 10 years ago, you may no longer be immune.

Several studies have suggested that a severe attack of flu early in pregnancy may increase the risk of miscarriage, but it may be as well not to take these results at face value. If a woman is asked whether she was ill when pregnant, she is more likely to recall an illness if problems arose with her pregnancy at a later date. This effect will be particularly marked with common and indistinct illnesses like flu. Many, perhaps most, women will suffer a flu-like illness at some time in pregnancy, but women who later miscarried are more likely to remember these illnesses.

There is no evidence that common childhood illnesses like measles or chickenpox cause miscarriage if caught during pregnancy, although there is a question mark over mumps, as one study suggested that mumps may sometimes infect the fetus and lead to miscarriage. The risk of miscarriage according to this study was doubled if the mother caught mumps.[9] Even if you are unlucky enough to catch mumps in early pregnancy, this still leaves you with a good chance of carrying the pregnancy to term.

Toxoplasma gondii is an organism found in cats' faeces which can cause miscarriage in humans. This is why pregnant women are advised to wear rubber gloves when gardening or cleaning out the cat litter — a simple enough precaution against a rather remote possibility.

About half of all women have mycoplasma bacteria in their cervices, and it has been suggested that these bacteria, especially the T-strain mycoplasma, may cause miscarriage. This seems unlikely, as there are so many infected women and most of them do not miscarry, but some doctors may treat women who have these bacteria with erythromycin (an antibiotic) before they become pregnant again or during pregnancy.

Endometriosis is recognized as a cause of infertility and may also occasionally cause miscarriage. In endometriosis, pieces of the endometrium or uterine lining become attached to other parts of the pelvic organs or the abdominal cavity. These patches of tissue continue to behave like the uterine lining, changing through the month and then bleeding during a period. As the menstrual flow cannot escape, inflammation and scar tissue result. About two-thirds of women with this condition have symptoms, including heavy periods, severe menstrual pain — often starting several days before a period — and severe pain on intercourse. Minor surgery seems to lead to a greatly improved chance of successful pregnancy in women with endometriosis. If you have had one or more miscarriages, and suspect you have endometriosis, you should discuss this with your doctor before you try for another pregnancy.

DRUGS

Certain medical drugs are known to cause birth defects and women are generally advised to avoid taking non-prescribed medical drugs during pregnancy. There is at present very little evidence that taking medical drugs in pregnancy may cause miscarriage, but this may be because there is so little research on the subject. One study did find an increased miscarriage rate among women sufferers from migraine, and among the wives of male migraine sufferers, which was attributed to the use of ergotamine preparations.[10]

Street drugs have also been associated with reproductive effects. For instance, marijuana may interfere with the development of sperm, heroin very often disrupts the menstrual cycle, and LSD may cause chromosomal damage. Where a number of other reproductive effects are found, it seems likely that there is also an increased risk of miscarriage.

CONTRACEPTION

Recently there has been a lot of publicity given to the temporary infertility suffered by some women when they come off the contraceptive pill. This has led some medical professionals to ask whether women who have taken the pill in the past are more likely to miscarry. But several studies have shown that oral contraceptives do not increase the risk of miscarriage, even in women who were taking the pill until the last period before conception. There may however be a slight increase in early miscarriage in those rare cases where a woman becomes pregnant while taking the pill.

Barrier methods (the cap, diaphragm or condom) do not increase the risk of miscarriage. This remains true even when you get pregnant while using one of these methods.

If a woman has an IUD removed and then gets pregnant, she is slightly more likely to have an ectopic pregnancy. But if, as sometimes happens, she gets pregnant with the IUD in place, she will have a one in two chance of miscarrying, probably after 12 weeks. Miscarriages with the IUD in place are caused by infection of the womb, and such infections pose a serious risk to the health of mother as well as baby. So, if you are unlucky enough to get pregnant while using the IUD, it is vital that you have the IUD removed as soon as possible, whether or not you want to continue the pregnancy.

INDUCED ABORTION

The woman who has had an abortion in the past may worry that this was the cause of her miscarriage. Studies done before 1975 suggested that induced abortions did increase the risk of miscarriage in subsequent pregnancies. Many of these miscarriages were caused by cervical incompetence, as the techniques of abortion used in the past sometimes damaged the cervix.

Since 1975, there has been considerable improvement in abortion methods. As a result, studies done in the past 10 years have found no link between previous abortion and miscarriage.

ENVIRONMENTAL HAZARDS

In 1985, an accident at the Union Carbide plant in Bhopal, India, led to the release of a cloud of the gas methyl isocyanate, and possibly of cyanide. More than 2,000 people were killed. Miscarriages and stillbirths were among the other early effects of the tragedy.

In 1979, people who lived in the Love Canal area of New York became concerned about health problems in their families. Many children were becoming seriously ill, and there seemed to be unusually high rates of miscarriage, stillbirth and birth defects in the community. It was discovered that the local school was built on top of a chemical graveyard. Metal drums containing chemical waste had rusted and the chemicals had been seeping out into the water supply and the soil.

In the late 1970s in Oregon, women discovered that they and their neighbours were suffering unusually high numbers of miscarriages, mostly in the spring. They discovered the miscarriages were happening in areas which had been sprayed with the herbicide 2,4,5,-T, which contains dioxin, one of the most poisonous chemicals known to man. Dioxin was an ingredient of Agent Orange, used to defoliate the Vietnamese countryside during the Vietnam war, and associated with miscarriages, stillbirths, birth defects and cancer among the Vietnamese and in the families of American soldiers.

In 1985, the Governor of California ordered an enquiry into a rise in the miscarriage rate in Silicon Valley in California. Women were suffering between two and three times as many miscarriages as would be predicted. It was found that water in the area had been contaminated when underground storage tanks belonging to one silicon-chip manufacturer leaked 60,000 gallons of toxic chemicals.

Research has suggested that the average American male today produces less than half the sperm produced by the average male fifty years ago. Flame retardants used to cut down the fire risks associated with foam mattresses have been blamed.[11]

Pollution must be a source of intense concern to everyone who thinks about the future, but especially, perhaps, to women. Women are more intimately involved than men with the welfare of children — not just the children already born, or the children about to be born, but also the children not yet conceived, the fantasy children of our imagined futures. It is women who carry the major burden of anxiety about the effects of pollution on those children.

This anxiety has a sound scientific basis. The fetus is the

most vulnerable human organism and may be damaged by doses of poisons that do not affect the health of adults, or that cause cancer or other illnesses in adults only after years of exposure. Any poison that harms the fetus could lead to a rise in the miscarriage rate. An abnormality in the fetus makes miscarriage more likely — the death of the fetus makes miscarriage inevitable.

It makes sense, then, to ask: could environmental hazards be causing some of our miscarriages? Could we be endangering our babies by drinking water that contains traces of industrial chemicals, or by walking through fields that have been sprayed with pesticides, or by living near toxic waste dumps or industrial plants that make toxic chemicals?

There is virtually no research that attempts to answer these questions. There are various reasons for the lack of research. Firstly, it is difficult to do. Studies of the relationship between illness and pollution are usually retrospective — they look back to past events — and so it is impossible to be sure of the exact degree of exposure to which people were subjected. Secondly, miscarriage is a hidden event. Where researchers look at the effects of pollution, they are more likely to look for problems like cancer or birth defects than a rise in the miscarriage rate. Even where researchers are concerned with miscarriage, early miscarriage is easily overlooked, because it takes place before the woman has attended the ante-natal clinic. Thirdly, and probably most important, there are vested interests. Research is funded either by government or industry. Industrialists themselves are unlikely to question their practice unless forced to do so. Governments are unwilling to fund research into the damage done by industrial pollution when the industry concerned is contributing to the Gross National Product. Such reluctance is disturbingly short-sighted. What could be of more importance to a society than the health of its children?

There are times when we may look at our polluted world and feel overwhelmed by the dangers to our children, both born and yet to be born. We may feel powerless and despairing.

If you are pregnant or planning pregnancy and feel this despair, remind yourself that at worst these hazards mean an increased risk. Even where women are exposed to known poisons, many babies will still be carried to term and be born healthy. By giving yourself some credits on the balance sheet, and in particular, by having as good a diet as possible, you may be able to do something to minimize the risk.

We can remind ourselves, too, that in the longer term, we are not entirely powerless. By sharing experiences of pregnancy problems, women and men may help to identify reproductive hazards in the environment. Miscarriage is not simply a private grief. The miscarriage rate may also be the most sensitive barometer of the health of a population.

SOURCES

Susan Borg and Judith Lasker, *When Pregnancy Fails*, RKP, London, 1982

Bob DeMatteo, *Terminal Shock*, NC Press Ltd, Toronto, 1986

John Elkington, *The Poisoned Womb*, Penguin, Harmondsworth, 1986

General, Municipal, Boilermakers' and Allied Trades Union, 'Your reproductive health at risk', April 1984

Hera Unit, 'Smoking in pregnancy — a review', The Spastics Society, 1982

Barry Stimmel (ed) *The effects of Maternal Alcohol and Drug Abuse on the Newborn*, Haworth Press, New York, 1982

REFERENCES

1. H.J. Huisjes, *Spontaneous Abortion*, Churchill Livingstone, Edinburgh, 1984, p. 39
2. Andrew Chetley, 'Dangerous pesticides', *New Internationalist*, March 1987, p. 27
3. DeMatteo, *op cit*, preface to second edition
4. S. Harlap and P.H. Shiono, 'Alcohol, smoking and incidence of spontaneous abortions in the first and second trimester', *The Lancet*, 26 July 1980, p. 173
5. J. Kline, P. Shrout, Z. Stein, M. Susser and D. Warburton, 'Drinking during pregnancy and spontaneous abortion', *The Lancet*, 26 July 1980, p. 176
6. F.M. Badr and R.S. Badr, 'Induction of dominant lethal mutation in male mice by ethyl alcohol', *Nature*, vol. 253, 10 January 1975, p. 134
7. J. Kline *et al*, 'Smoking: a risk factor for spontaneous abortion', *New England Journal of Medicine*, vol. 297, no. 15, 13 October 1977, p. 793
8. Evans *et al*, 'Sperm abnormalities and cigarette smoking.' *The Lancet*, 21 March 1981, p. 627
9. Huisjes, *op cit*, p. 117
10. Huisjes, *op cit*, p. 106
11. Elkington, *op cit*, p. 48

4.
TESTS AND TREATMENTS

I have had my chances. I have tried and tried.
I have stitched life into me like a rare organ.
And walked carefully, precariously, like something rare.
I have tried not to think too hard. I have tried to be
natural.
SYLVIA PLATH, *Three Women*

After my miscarriage, I became convinced there was something wrong with my body. Plainly I was not a proper woman — otherwise why would the miscarriage have happened? Obviously something was missing, or something was not working properly.

This belief that your body is in some way defective is very common following a miscarriage. Fortunately most of the time, this belief is wrong. Most women who miscarry have reproductive systems in perfect working order and the problem lies with the arrangement of chromosomes in the fetus, or in the ovum or sperm.

However, for certain women, there are problems in the way their bodies are put together, or in the way they work, and these women are more likely than the rest of the population to miscarry. Some of them suffer the distress of recurrent miscarriage. A number of these conditions can be identified by tests, and, for some, treatment is now available.

HORMONE DEFICIENCY

One of the most persistent theories about recurrent miscarriage has put the blame on low levels of female sex hormones. When treatment has been based on this theory, women have had their hormone levels boosted with injections, tablets or suppositories containing various hormones.

Hormones are powerful substances and can affect the

workings of the body in unpredictable ways. The story of DES shows that doctors are wise to be cautious about the use of hormone treatment. DES (diethylstilboestrol) was a synthetic substitute for oestrogen, used in the 1950s and 1960s as a treatment for miscarriage. Some daughters of the treated women developed rare cancers, and many had abnormalities of their reproductive organs which made them more likely to suffer miscarriage themselves. It is a terrible irony that a treatment for miscarriage has led to a greater risk of miscarriage for the daughters of those pregnancies. DES treatment was stopped in most countries by 1971.

Nowadays, when hormone treatment is offered to women who have suffered recurrent miscarriage, the hormone in question is usually progesterone. As progesterone is made by the corpus luteum, inadequate progesterone production is also called corpus luteum deficiency.

The efficiency of the corpus luteum can be tested when the woman is not pregnant. Progesterone levels in her blood and urine are measured and a sample of tissue (biopsy) is taken from the endometrium (the lining of the womb) and analysed in the laboratory to see how well it has grown. If the endometrium is not as mature as it should be, this will suggest the woman's progesterone levels are low. It may be concluded that it is progesterone deficiency which is causing her to miscarry. The woman may also be asked to take her temperature each morning as the temperature goes up in response to progesterone production. It does seem, however, that doctors quite frequently prescribe progesterone treatment without doing any tests first. This is unwise, because inappropriate hormone treatment may prolong a pregnancy that is going to fail anyway, a situation that is clearly best avoided. Treatment may be by suppositories inserted into the vagina or rectum, or by injections. The dosage, and the length of time treatment is continued, vary greatly according to the practice of different doctors.

There is disagreement within the medical profession about the usefulness of this treatment. It has so far been impossible to prove that corpus luteum deficiency actually causes miscarriage. Women who are about to miscarry do have low progesterone levels, but this proves nothing — lowering of hormone levels is an effect rather than the cause of the miscarriage. However some studies have shown that a few women who have suffered miscarriages have somewhat lower than normal progesterone levels when they are not pregnant. This suggests that progesterone deficiency might be playing a part in their miscarriages.

After her first baby, Sue had two 'missed miscarriages' at 16 weeks and at 12 weeks. When her fourth pregnancy was confirmed at five weeks she was offered hormone treatment:

> The injections were given by the community midwives who came to the house every Tuesday and Friday. At first the jabs made me slightly woozy, but by week seven I began to feel very sick about three hours after the jab and had to go to bed or lie down by tea time. The next day I was less nauseous and just ate less than usual. The only other ill-effect I suffered was an inflamed itchy patch around the injection site on alternate buttocks. We decided this was due to the technique of some of the midwives, as it only happened occasionally. It was avoided by giving two jabs for the two hormones and by vigorous rubbing of the site after the jab to disperse the hormone. By 13 weeks the ill-effects had all gone and the treatment was stopped after a successful 16-week scan.

UTERINE ABNORMALITIES

Some women are born with abnormally shaped wombs. There are a number of different abnormalities possible. Some women have a septum — a wall of membrane — running down the middle of the uterus, others may have a double uterus, or a bicornuate (two-horned) uterus. For women who have uterine

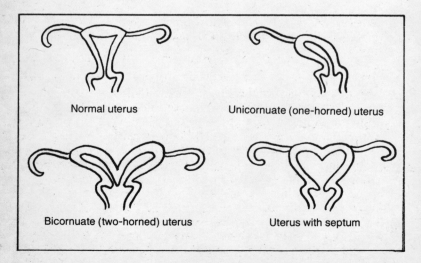

FIGURE 3 Some uterine abnormalities

abnormalities there is an increased risk of miscarriage both before and after 14 weeks. No-one knows how common uterine abnormalities are, but it has been suggested they may affect 1 in 100 women. Women whose mothers were treated with DES when they themselves were pregnant are particularly likely to have uterine abnormalities.

It has been estimated that uterine abnormalities may account for anything between 8 per cent and 30 per cent of recurrent miscarriages. It is not entirely understood why there is this increased risk. One theory has been that there simply is not enough space in the abnormally shaped womb for the growing baby. Other doctors maintain that it is not that simple, as markedly abnormal wombs are sometimes able to accommodate a growing fetus. Consultant obstetrician Dr Gillian Lachelin[1] comments, 'I have even delivered normal healthy twins from a woman with a completely bicornuate [two-horned] uterus — there was a baby in each uterine horn.' Another possibility is that the placenta may implant on a part of the uterus which does not have an adequate blood supply to nourish the fetus. Also some of the miscarriages suffered by women with abnormal wombs may be caused by cervical incompetence, as women with abnormal wombs have an increased chance that the cervix will not work properly.

Diagnosis is usually made by hysterosalpingogram. This is an X-ray test in which a contrast dye that will show up on X-ray is injected into the womb and Fallopian tubes. The X-ray will be done within 10 days of the start of a period to ensure the woman is not pregnant, as X-rays can harm the fetus.

Debbie was given a hysterosalpingogram as part of the investigations after her third miscarriage:

On arrival at the clinic I was given a hospital gown and asked to empty my bladder. I was then asked to lie flat on the X-ray table with my bottom and feet at the end, knees bent up, while the radiologist sat at the foot of the table. First he swabbed me, then he proceeded to insert a variety of instruments into my vagina. The last of these was an enormous looking syringe-type object, which contained the dye. The long nozzle on this had to be passed through my cervix into the uterus, and despite having been told this would be a fairly painless procedure I had a sudden severe period-type pain which subsided a little once the instrument was in place. Then I was heaved back along the table by my shoulders so that I was lying flat with my legs out straight, all ready to be X-rayed. On a small screen I could see what was inside of me. The dye was injected in and revealed the shape

of my uterus and tubes. My mind was taken off my
discomfort a little by the weird-looking shape of the uterus on
the screen. In fact I do have a bicornuate uterus, but I was
told I should discuss the implications of this with my
consultant.

The whole procedure was over in about 10 to 15 minutes
and I was told after resting a minute to go to the toilet and
strain to expel the dye. The pain I had experienced lessened
considerably once the syringe had been removed. There was a
little bleeding afterwards and I had a fairly severe period-
type pain for several hours accompanied by backache.

Debbie has since learned that other women have also been
promised a painless experience, but have in fact found
themselves in quite a lot of pain.

If your uterus is found on X-ray to be abnormal, you may be
offered surgery. The decision about whether to accept surgery is
not a simple one. The operation leaves scarring on the uterus,
and as a result up to 30 per cent of women who have this form of
surgery may become infertile.[2] This is a very high risk, although
for a woman who has already experienced a number of
miscarriages, it may be an acceptable one. After discussing the
options with her consultant, Debbie decided against surgery.
Her fourth and fifth pregnancies were both successful.

It is important to note that a hysterosalpingogram, like any
other invasive procedure, does carry a slight risk of infection.
After a hysterosalpingogram, you should contact your doctor
immediately if you have any of the following symptoms: pain
that lasts longer than a few hours, very severe pain, or fever.

FIBROIDS

Fibroids are non-malignant growths in the muscle of the uterine
wall. They are extremely common, especially in women over 30,
while at least one in five women over 40 have them. At one time
they were regarded as a possible cause of recurrent miscarriage,
but medical opinion has since changed and fibroids are no
longer seen as a possible cause of miscarriage.

However, some kinds of fibroids, in particular fibroids that
protrude into the uterine cavity, can cause problems later in
pregnancy. If it is found that you have such a fibroid, you may
be offered surgery to have it removed.

CERVICAL INCOMPETENCE

The term 'cervical incompetence' refers to a malfunction of the cervix, the neck of the womb. In a miscarriage caused by cervical incompetence, the cervix is unable to hold the contents of the womb (the fetus, placenta and bag of waters) in place. The cervix dilates (opens) much too early allowing the baby to be expelled before it is fully developed and able to survive. This problem probably accounts for between 1 in 10 and 1 in 5 of all miscarriages that take place after 14 weeks of pregnancy. Most often they take place between the 16th and 24th weeks.

Medical textbooks describe the characteristic features of a miscarriage caused by cervical incompetence as follows: there is little or no bleeding before the waters break, although there may be an increase in the normal vaginal mucous discharge. The woman's waters will break quite quickly. There may be little or no pain and the baby is pushed out in just a few contractions. The baby has not died in the womb and has no chromosomal defects.

This is described as the 'typical' picture, but it is possible that there may be degrees of cervical incompetence. There may be late miscarriages that do not quite fit this picture — perhaps with more bleeding or pain — but weakness of the cervix may still be the suspected cause.

Although it is not known exactly what causes cervical incompetence, there are clues in the histories of women with this problem. Many of these women have suffered some kind of surgical damage to the cervix. In other words, cervical incompetence is often an 'iatrogenic' or doctor-induced condition. A cone biopsy, an operation in which pre-cancerous tissue is cut away from the cervix, might cause this damage. So might a forceful dilatation and curettage (D & C) in which the cervix is excessively dilated. There is no need to worry if you have had a routine D & C, perhaps after a previous miscarriage. It is also unlikely that the cervix would have been weakened by an induced abortion done in recent years, although some women have had their cervices damaged by induced abortions done in or before the early 1970s, before the risks of excessive dilatation were recognized. A very difficult birth can also occasionally damage the cervix — if for instance a large baby is born very rapidly before the cervix is fully dilated, or if there is a difficult forceps delivery before the cervix is fully dilated.

Occasionally, women are born with cervical incompetence. It is found in women who have uterine abnormalities, and in women who were exposed to the drug DES when in the womb themselves. It is also possible that the condition may be inherited.

The treatment for cervical incompetence is called the cervical stitch. It is just what it says — a stitch put in the cervix that closes the internal os and prevents it from dilating. It is one form of treatment for miscarriage which seems to be extremely effective.

Ros Kane, a journalist who herself gave birth to a daughter after having a cervical stitch, carried out a survey of 146 women who had received this treatment. Surveys of women's experiences of miscarriage suggest that women are much more likely to recall bad experiences of treatment than good ones, but this survey of experiences with the cervical stitch produced a very different response. The vast majority of the women were delighted with the treatment. Most were convinced, after their previous experiences of one or more late miscarriages, that they could not have had their babies without it.

There are two kinds of stitches — the Shirodkar and the MacDonald — called after the doctors who invented them. Both use a tape which, unlike the material used in most medical stitching, cannot be absorbed by the body. The tape is inserted round the cervix at the level of the internal os, preventing it from opening. The stitch may be put in before you become pregnant, or, more usually, during pregnancy, most often at about 14 weeks, after the time for early miscarriage caused for instance by chromosomal defects has passed. The stitch is usually put in under general anaesthetic. You will have to stay in bed for at least 24 hours after the stitch has been inserted, and you will probably be kept in hospital for several days. Half the women in Ros Kane's survey felt no pain afterwards, while the rest had some pain, which ranged from a 'slight ache' to 'painful tummy for ages'.

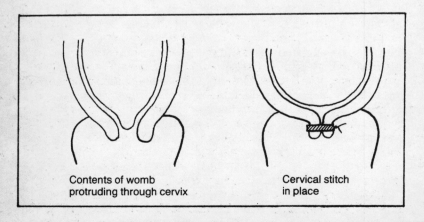

Contents of womb
protruding through cervix

Cervical stitch
in place

FIGURE 4 Cervical incompetence

If you are already pregnant and have an incompetent cervix and have not had a stitch, the problem may show up on a scan after about 11 weeks. The internal os will be much wider than it would be in a woman with a normal cervix. Some women with this problem in pregnancy get a feeling of heaviness or pressure in the vagina, as the membranes start to bulge through the cervix as it dilates. If the problem only comes to light in pregnancy, when the waters have already started to leak, it may still be possible to have a stitch.

Some women are aware of the stitch, especially towards the end of the pregnancy. One woman for instance, described a feeling like a pin being stuck into her. Many women stress the importance of resting as much as possible during pregnancy, making comments like 'Rest as soon as you feel pulling or aching'. It is quite common to have increased yellow or white vaginal discharge due to the stitch. You should mention this to your doctor, particularly if it becomes smelly, as a severe discharge may indicate that you have an infection of the cervix caused by the stitch. If left untreated, an infection could itself lead to miscarriage.

It is essential that the stitch be removed if you start to miscarry or when labour starts, as otherwise there is a risk that the womb will rupture. If you have a stitch, you should contact your doctor immediately if you have any vaginal bleeding, leakage of fluid or contractions.

If labour has not yet started, the stitch is removed at about 38 weeks of pregnancy. The doctor first puts in a speculum, so he can see the cervix. He finds the ends, snips the knots and pulls the stitch out. The procedure sounds simple enough, and it is not normally done under anaesthetic, but removal of the stitch can be very painful. This is particularly likely if your cervix is high, or if the stitch was inserted high up. Removal may also be painful if the stitch has become embedded, something that is more likely to happen if the stitch was put in before conception. It is therefore a good idea to ask your doctor what pain relief will be available.

Research suggests that when the stitch is put in early there is an 80 to 90 per cent success rate. If the stitch is put in after the woman has started to bleed or once the cervix has started to dilate or the bag of waters has pushed down into the vagina, the success rate is much lower, but the procedure may still be successful.

So here we have an effective treatment without too many risks to the mother or baby. Yet the doctor who advocates it has a dilemma: when should it be used? There is no generally accepted test for cervical incompetence. This means that diagnosis is usually made on the history of the previous miscarriage, in other words the problem will not come to light until the woman has suffered the intense distress of one or more late miscarriages. It also means that doctors vary enormously in their rates of treatment. Some obstetricians make little use of the stitch, or even question whether the diagnosis 'cervical incompetence' has any validity.

The lack of a definite diagnosis can sap the woman's confidence. Pamela had a miscarriage at 21 weeks. In some respects her miscarriage did not follow the typical pattern that the medical textbooks describe. She commented, 'They say next time I'll have a stitch put in and it'll be all right. How can they be so sure? They don't even know for certain what caused it, so how can they know it's going to be all right next time?'

In spite of the dilemma about when it should be used, the cervical stitch still remains one of the few treatments for miscarriage which gets a big vote of confidence from the women who have experienced it for themselves.

IMMUNOLOGICAL PROBLEMS

Immunological treatment is a new form of treatment for recurrent miscarriage. The first trials of this treatment were carried out at St Mary's Hospital, London, but the treatment is now being offered in some other centres. A recent study suggests that immunological treatment is very effective for a particular group of women. In a series of 113 pregnancies in women who had suffered recurrent miscarriages in the past, and who were screened and found suitable for this treatment, there were 89 successful deliveries. Yet just how this treatment works is still not entirely understood.[3]

The immune system is the mechanism by which the body defends itself against foreign and possibly harmful substances. You can see the immune system in action when you get an infected cut on your finger. The redness and swelling that appear are caused by the immune system fighting off the infection. It is the immune system, too, that causes the rise in your temperature if you catch flu. And it is because of the immune system that transplanted organs are rejected, unless the patient is treated with medication that suppresses the immune response. In all these situations, the immune system is identifying and attempting to reject or destroy foreign objects that might be harmful.

The bundle of cells that forms in the mother's Fallopian tubes after fertilization, and that then moves down and implants in the uterus, is in a sense a foreign object, for it is the father's genes that give some of this material its genetic instructions. You would therefore expect the mother's body immediately to reject this foreign material, but in normal pregnancy this does not happen. The chain of events is thought to be something like this. The tissue of the embryo contains substances called antigens from the father, and it is these antigens that alert the mother's body to the fact that this tissue is foreign. In response to the antigens, the mother produces substances called antibodies. These act as protection for the baby and are vital if the pregnancy is to succeed. The antibodies stop the expected rejection of foreign material from occurring and the baby, although different from the mother, is not miscarried.

Sometimes the mother's body fails to produce antibodies. If this happens, she will have recurrent miscarriages. And if, as occasionally happens, a woman with few or no antibodies to her partner does carry a baby to term there is a higher than normal risk that the baby will not grow properly in the womb.

A woman who has been pregnant at some time in the past will normally still have antibodies to her partner in her blood, antibodies that were stimulated by the previous pregnancy. Some women who have had recurrent miscarriages have been found not to have any antibodies to their partners. It is these women who respond to immunological treatment.

There are different theories about why the mother may fail to produce these crucial antibodies. One theory is that this happens where the parents resemble each other too closely. According to this theory, it is the 'foreignness' of the baby that stimulates the mother's body to produce the antibodies, so if the man and woman are genetically similar, for instance if they are relatives, the production of antibodies is not stimulated, and the baby is at some point rejected and miscarried. If this is the case, the woman might have no difficulty carrying a pregnancy by another man to term. However some researchers have found that couples suffering from recurrent miscarriages and helped by immunology treatment did not have more antigens in common than would be expected from random mating. Another theory is that there is something wrong with the actual process by which the mother's cells 'recognize' the embryo as foreign.

Whatever the explanation, the treatment seems to work for many couples. Treatment involves immunizing the woman against her partner by injections of white blood cells taken from his blood. Blood is taken from the man, and the white cells are separated, washed, suspended in medium, and then injected into the woman. In response to the injection, the woman makes the missing protective factor which will prevent her rejecting the embryo.

Media stories about immunological treatment have raised many women's hopes that at last something can be done to help them, but only certain women will be considered suitable, even for testing. For instance, at St Mary's, women are only tested if they have had three or more miscarriages and no more than one pregnancy beyond 28 weeks.[4] However because the theory on which treatment is based is about an interaction between the woman and her partner, only pregnancies by your present partner are counted. In other words, if you have had two children with a previous partner, and three miscarriages with your present partner, you could still be considered for treatment. Women who have had one or two miscarriages are excluded because statistically they have as good a chance of having a successful pregnancy next time without treatment as with it. And women who in addition to their miscarriages have had two or more pregnancies which have progressed beyond 28 weeks are excluded, as they have been found not to benefit from treatment.

If you come into the group of suitable women and are referred to St Mary's, blood will be taken from both of you and tested, to see whether the woman has antibodies to her partner. It can be extremely disappointing to come this far, and then to be told that your antibody levels are normal and you will not be offered treatment.

Julia had one son, then three miscarriages. She was tested and found to be suitable for immunology treatment. After the treatment, Julia felt optimistic. 'I had a huge lump on my arm, so obviously I was reacting to my husband's blood cells.' But there were doubts, too, particularly as the treatment was so new, for Julia was part of the original trial. 'They say this is the right thing, but you wonder, is it really? I wondered — was I miscarrying because my babies weren't properly formed? Was there something else wrong? As the pregnancy got near to term, I thought, it's got so far, but is it going to last long enough? Would the antibodies see me through the whole pregnancy?' Fortunately the treatment did see her through and her baby daughter was born at term.

Looking back, Julia commented, 'The amazing thing was, how simple it was. Everything else seems to be so hit and miss — they'd say, "Well, we might try this, we might try that." It was incredible to find somebody who said, "Look, this is your problem."'

FERTILITY PROBLEMS AND MISCARRIAGE

Couples who have difficulty in conceiving have a slightly higher risk of miscarriage than the rest of the population.

Jill started trying for a baby at 34. After a year she was referred to an Infertility Clinic, prescribed Clomid, an ovulation-inducing drug, and put on a waiting list for a laparoscopy (an operation in which the ovaries, tubes and uterus are viewed through a lighted telescope).

> The following month I missed a period. I had no pregnancy symptoms and two pregnancy tests produced negative results. Hormone levels must have been low, and my pregnancy was not confirmed until I was 9 weeks pregnant. At 11 weeks I started to bleed, and at 12 weeks I lost my baby.
>
> At first despite the pain and grief which followed my miscarriage I felt at least I now had hope for the future. The doctors at the clinic were very encouraging. No need for a laparoscopy now, they said. If I got pregnant once, I was bound to do so again. Well, it's now over a year since my miscarriage. I have not conceived again and after nearly two years the clinic has still failed to find any reason why.

No-one understands why the woman who takes a long time to conceive is more likely than other women to miscarry. However it is easy enough to speculate about possible links between infertility and miscarriage, as both may have the same underlying cause. For instance, a woman with hormonal problems may take a long time to conceive because her cycle is irregular, and may also have difficulty in holding on to pregnancies. If a man has a low sperm count he may have fertility problems, and he may also have a higher proportion of abnormal sperm, so if his partner does conceive there may be a higher risk of miscarriage. It is also possible that apparently infertile women are actually conceiving and having very early recurrent miscarriages.

Couples with fertility problems who also suffer miscarriages have a double source of distress. It can be heartbreaking to try for a baby, perhaps for several years, then be thrilled to find yourself pregnant, only to have your hopes brought crashing down when you miscarry.

You may be wondering if you have a fertility problem. To give you some idea, here are some statistics from Dr Andrew Stanway's book *Why Us?*:[5]

In a couple making love on an unrestricted basis, the average time to conception is 5.3 months. 25% of couples will have conceived in the first month, 63% by the end of 6 months, 75% by the end of 9 months and 80% by the end of a year. A further 10% will have conceived by 18 months.

Most doctors will start investigating the problem if you have been trying for between 12 and 18 months.

It is estimated that about half of all infertile couples can be helped by medical treatment. Unfortunately most forms of infertility treatment are also associated with a slightly higher than normal miscarriage rate.

After miscarriage, many women think, 'What if I never even get pregnant again?' So remember that, although there is a link between miscarriage and infertility, this only affects a small group of women. The fact that you have miscarried does not affect your chances of conceiving in the future. If you conceived without too much difficulty last time, there is no reason why you should not conceive easily again.

HYDATIDIFORM MOLE (MOLAR PREGNANCY)

Hydatidiform mole is a rare kind of abnormal pregnancy that may produce symptoms of threatened miscarriage. The problem is believed to arise when an 'empty' ovum — that is one which lacks the essential genetic material — is fertilized by a normal sperm.

In a hydatidiform mole, the placenta grows very fast, producing a mass of cysts that look rather like a bunch of grapes, hence the name, as 'hydatid' means 'watery cyst'. As the rapid growth of the placenta raises the woman's hormone levels, she may experience severe nausea and vomiting, and may develop high blood pressure too. Her womb may be disproportionately large for the stage of pregnancy. She may have vaginal bleeding, sometimes very dark, described as 'prune-coloured'.

Molar pregnancies are on average diagnosed at about 16 weeks. They show up clearly on an ultrasound scan — the picture looks like a snowstorm. The woman would miscarry eventually, but the pregnancy will be terminated immediately, usually by suction aspiration under general anaesthetic. This must be done even when the woman has already miscarried, to make sure that her uterus is completely empty.

If any tissue from the mole remains in the womb, it may continue to grow and become cancerous. This cancer, called choriocarcinoma, is virtually 100 per cent curable if it is caught in time. Because of this risk, women who have had a hydatidiform mole are given frequent checkups in the months following the pregnancy. Any problems can be easily detected, for if molar tissue is still growing in the womb, there will be raised levels of the hormone HCG (human chorionic gonadotrophin) in the woman's blood and urine.

In the past women were told to wait two years before getting pregnant again, because of the risk of cancer. Some doctors still advise this. Other doctors nowadays may suggest women try again sooner — perhaps after six months or one year — if their test results are normal.

A woman who has already had a mole has a 1 in 50 risk of having another. There is also a slight tendency for them to run in families. However, even if you have had two successive molar pregnancies, you still have a good chance of having a normal pregnancy next time.

The aftermath of a molar pregnancy may present particular difficulties for women. As it is so rare, women often have not heard of it and the need for information is pressing. Then there is the frightening possibility of developing cancer. As Chris remarked, 'I was absolutely devastated not only to lose my baby but to learn I had something like this. I was convinced I was going to die of cancer and even though the consultant explained gently that I was just to try and put it to the back of my mind and be patient, I can't seem to accept it.'

Having to wait to get pregnant again may feel unbearable. Louise remembers, 'I found out from a nurse in a very matter-of-fact way that I'd have to wait two years before I could try again. I was devastated.' In fact, if the tests are normal for several months, you may be advised that it is safe for you to try again. Louise asked if she could get pregnant again after 12 months, and was told that she could. In her next pregnancy, she had some bleeding at 8 weeks. She rushed to hospital and demanded a scan. This showed that the baby was still alive. The bleeding stopped and she went on to give birth to a healthy baby.

ECTOPIC PREGNANCY

If you have had an ectopic pregnancy, you will have known about it, and you will probably have had abdominal surgery. So this section will not help you to think about possible causes for your miscarriage or miscarriages, but there are two reasons for including this condition here. One reason is that ectopic pregnancy can be confused with a miscarriage, as the most likely symptoms are pain and bleeding. The other is that it is one of the most dangerous complications of pregnancy and it is therefore important that women should be aware of this possibility.

Ectopic means 'out-of-place'. In normal conception, the bundle of cells, once fertilized, moves down the Fallopian tube into the womb and implants in the lining of the womb. In an ectopic pregnancy, however the bundle of cells implants in some other place — most probably in one of the Fallopian tubes, which is why it is sometimes called tubal pregnancy, although it might also be in one of the ovaries or in the abdominal cavity. Some ectopic pregnancies give a positive reading on a pregnancy test, others do not. There may be some of the signs of early pregnancy, such as missed periods, nausea, breast tenderness, although these are by no means always present. Most women with ectopic pregnancies experience some vaginal bleeding.

An ectopic pregnancy is difficult to diagnose. An ultrasound scan will show that the uterus is empty, and where this picture is combined with symptoms of pregnancy there are obvious grounds for suspecting that the pregnancy is ectopic. Unfortunately the scan cannot show what is happening outside the womb, nor is it possible to diagnose an ectopic pregnancy by an internal examination. Occasionally the woman will complain of shoulder pain. This is referred pain — pain that is caused by a problem in one part of the body but is felt in another. Shoulder pain is a rare symptom, but when it is present, it makes the diagnosis much easier.

FIGURE 5 Two common sites for an ectopic pregnancy

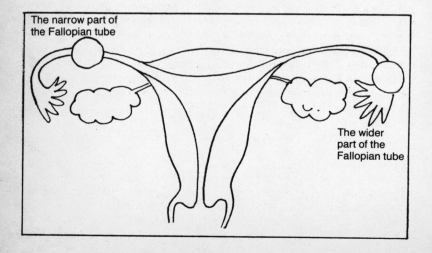

The narrow part of the Fallopian tube

The wider part of the Fallopian tube

The Fallopian tube may eventually burst, between about 8 and 12 weeks of pregnancy. This sometimes occurs when the woman is straining to have a bowel movement. The pain may be agonizing and the woman may go into shock from acute loss of blood. This is a medical emergency and requires immediate surgery. Alternatively, if the fertilized cell has implanted in a wider part of the tube, the rupture of the tube may be gradual causing intermittent bleeding and pain that starts and stops, more like a threatened miscarriage. When the tube bursts, whether this happens suddenly or slowly, the embryo will die and will be re-absorbed into the mother's body.

If your doctor suspects you may have an ectopic pregnancy, you will be admitted to hospital for a laparoscopy. Under general anaesthesia, the abdominal cavity is inflated slightly with carbon dioxide and a lighted telescope is inserted through a tiny incision in the navel. This allows the doctor to examine the uterus, Fallopian tubes and ovaries. The embryo is then removed through a small incision in the lower abdomen (a laparotomy). Nowadays every effort is made to preserve as much of the Fallopian tube and ovary as possible for future pregnancies, but even so the whole tube may have to be removed. However, even if a woman does lose a Fallopian tube this way, there is no reason why she cannot go on to have a subsequent normal pregnancy.

The causes of ectopic pregnancy are not clear, but it is known that previous pelvic infection (for example pelvic inflammatory disease) may make ectopic pregnancy more likely, because it may impair the ability of the Fallopian tube to conduct the fertilized ovum into the uterus. It is also known that use of an IUD increases the risk of ectopic pregnancy — women who have IUDs in place are ten times more likely than other women to have ectopic pregnancies. An IUD will stop an embryo from implanting normally in the womb, but it will not stop a pregnancy from implanting in the wrong place, in one of the tubes or in the ovary. Women who have fertility problems but whose tubes are quite normal also have an increased risk of ectopic pregnancy.

BALANCED TRANSLOCATION

If you have an early miscarriage, a chromosomal abnormality is the most likely cause. In fact between 50 and 60 per cent of fetuses that are miscarried before 12 weeks have chromosomal defects. However just because this has happened once does not make it any more likely that it will happen again. There is one kind of chromosomal problem, however, which does run the risk of being repeated. Occasionally, there is a permanent fault in one of the parent's sex cells — the cells in the ovaries or sperm. This defect is called a 'balanced translocation'. It is 'balanced' because there is the right amount of chromosomal material in total in the cell — all the genes are there — but some of them are permanently in the wrong place: there has been a 'movement across', a trans-location. If a person's sex cells have such a defect, he or she will produce a regular and fairly high proportion of abnormal ova or sperm. No-one knows how common these defects are although some experts think they may explain 1 in 20 recurrent miscarriages.

There is a fairly simple test for inherited chromosomal problems. Blood is taken from the parent and some of the cells are stained and examined under the microscope to establish the arrangement, number and size of the chromosomes. If tests show that either of you has a translocation, you will be given genetic counselling. The kind of damage to the fetus that might be caused by the translocation will be described to you, and you will be told the statistical likelihood of this damage recurring in future pregnancies. Different translocations involve different risks. When you next become pregnant you will be offered amniocentesis at about 16 weeks.

Sharon and her husband Paul had genetic testing after Sharon's third miscarriage, and Sharon was found to have a 'translocation of the 13/14th chromosome'. As Sharon explained:

> In simple terms this means, although I've no obvious defects, I'm a carrier and my chances of having a normal child are only 1 in 4. So if the babies I'd been carrying had gone to term, there's every chance they would've been abnormal — so my body had rejected them. The problems caused by my translocation include webbing of fingers, and heart and lung problems. So maybe we'd been lucky I'd not given birth to a child with one of these problems.
>
> We went home and talked long and hard about what to do. We both adore children and desperately wanted one of our own, but could we face the possibility of a handicapped one? Although he desperately wanted children, Paul knew the way these miscarriages were affecting me. It was my body which suffered, he pointed out, and he couldn't put me through it again and again, unless I was really sure.

Eventually for Sharon the decision formed itself. As so often with these excruciating decisions, a little thing happened that tipped the balance and clarified for her what she wanted to do.

'I came across an article in a woman's magazine, about a woman who had 13 miscarriages before having a baby. That did it. Until then, although I'd heard of lots of people having had miscarriages, it was always between children — not before.'

Sharon got pregnant again only to have another miscarriage. She and Paul decided to try just once more. Happily this, her fifth pregnancy, was successful and Matthew was born.

AMNIOCENTESIS

If tests show you or your partner to have a balanced translocation, you will be offered amniocentesis in your next pregnancy. In some health authorities, you may also be offered amniocentesis if you are over 35, as the risk of having a baby with Down's Syndrome starts to rise at this age. If an abnormality shows up, you will be offered an abortion.

Amniocentesis involves taking a sample of the water (amniotic fluid) that surrounds the baby in the uterus. A pool of fluid will be located using ultrasound. The mother's abdominal wall is numbed with a local anaesthetic injection, then a needle is inserted through the abdominal wall and a small amount of fluid is sucked out. The fluid is taken to the laboratory for analysis.

Amniocentesis is also used to test for spina bifida. It is offered to women whose blood samples have an unusually high level of alpha-fetoprotein. If the baby does have a neural tube defect the level of alpha-fetoprotein in the amniotic fluid will also be raised, confirming the suspicions aroused by the blood test. One in four women with abnormal blood tests do have babies with spina bifida.

Many women are grateful for amniocentesis. If it shows that nothing is wrong, you can have real peace of mind for the rest of the pregnancy. However the procedure is not without its risk and problems. The test itself is quite difficult to do. Occasionally it may require more than one attempt to obtain a sample of fluid, and even if fluid is obtained, the tests may not always give a reliable result. There is a small margin of error, so false results may be obtained. If an abnormality is present, it does not show the degree of handicap. This is not relevant in the case of chromosomal abnormalities, such as Down's Syndrome, but in the case of spina bifida, there are degrees of handicap and the level of abnormality may be only slight. The chromosome tests take about three to four weeks, so you are about 19 to 20 weeks pregnant by the time you get the results, and if they show something wrong you have to decide whether to have an abortion at a point when the baby is quite highly developed. And amniocentesis does itself involve a small risk of miscarriage — between 1 in 100 and 1 in 200 babies who are tested will miscarry as a result of the test.

Some of these difficulties may well be avoided by a new kind of test, at present being researched. In this test, called a chorion biopsy, tissue is taken via the vagina from the placental membrane, or chorion, that surrounds the fetus. Chorion biopsy has the obvious advantage that it can be done early in pregnancy. However this technique is still in its early stages of development, and at present has a higher risk of miscarriage associated with it, so as yet amniocentesis remains the only tested option.

The offer of amniocentesis presents you with two tough decisions. First there is the decision about whether to have the test at all, in view of the risk of miscarriage. Second there is the knowledge that you will have to make an excruciating decision if the results of the test show an abnormality.

Some doctors will only offer amniocentesis to couples who are willing to have an abortion if the baby is abnormal. Consultant obstetrician Dr Peter Huntingford comments,[6]

> I do not believe that you should ever be asked to consent to amniocentesis only if you agree to have the pregnancy terminated if the baby is found to be abnormal. ... None of us actually know what we would do — we may think that we do, but if the time ever came to make an actual decision we would probably surprise others, if not ourselves.

Linda and Mark had been through three miscarriages. In Linda's fourth pregnancy, she was given amniocentesis in view of her age — she was 38. The test was done at 18 weeks of pregnancy. Then she was contacted by the hospital and told that they could not get a result from the test. So Linda and Mark had to go to the hospital to discuss whether another test should be done.

Linda said,

> I had another scan. Mark and I watched our 21-week-old baby kick around. We saw perfect hands and feet, a small face with a mouth that kept opening and shutting. The baby's position was ideal for another test, but could we take the risk of damaging or even killing what was possibly a perfect child?
>
> We were left alone for about twenty minutes. I leaned on the windowsill, watching the red double-deckers crawling along Tottenham Court Road, seeing women shopping,

someone hailing a taxi — an ordinary day, out there. In my mind I ticked off the points. At our ages there is a higher risk of Down's Syndrome. Could we wait until June to find out if everything was all right? But I had nearly miscarried — was it fair to tamper with nature again? On the other hand, to go through all that sickness and worry and then — in the consultant's words — to 'get a dud'.

At the back of it all something was telling me to have faith in the baby, not to run any more risks, but just to let it grow in peace. I turned from the window to tell Mark what I'd thought and at the same moment he turned to me and said, very quietly, 'I think we should put on our coats and go home.'

We thanked everybody and did just that. In five minutes we were standing in the street, feeling relieved and strong in our decision. Now we would always believe that we had done the best that we could at the time.

Mark looked along the street for a taxi.

'Not yet,' I said. 'Let's just pop into Mothercare and have a look.'

'Great idea,' said Mark.

And we've been thinking positively ever since.

In this chapter I have described a number of different tests and treatments. Any offer of testing or treatment confronts you with a dilemma, the same dilemma that Linda and Mark had to face. Your doctor will advise you, but in the end the decision is yours. We can learn from Linda's story how these difficult decisions are often made.

Like Linda, you may hunt around for information. You may weigh up all the known facts — there may not be very many. You may despair of ever reaching a decision. Then, perhaps quite suddenly, you find that you know what you want to do. It is more like an intuition than a culmination of a process of thought. Sometimes it may go against the apparent logic of the situation. For Linda it was 'something telling me to have faith in the baby'. For another woman in another situation, it might be a different kind of feeling — a fear that something is indeed wrong, or a wish to go ahead with risky treatment.

Linda and Mark were fortunate. Twenty weeks later, their healthy daughter was born.

SOURCES

L.R. Curtis, G.B. Curtis, and M.K. Beard, *My Body — My Decision!*, HP Books Inc., Tucson, 1986

Peter Huntingford, *Birth Right*, BBC, London, 1985

H.J. Huisjes, *Spontaneous Abortion*, Churchill Livingstone, Edinburgh, 1984

Ros Kane, 'The cervical stitch: what it's like', The Miscarriage Association, 1986

Andrew Stanway, *Why Us?*, Thorsons, Wellingborough, 1984

REFERENCES

1. Gillian C.L. Lachelin, *Miscarriage, The Facts*, Oxford University Press, 1985
2. Huisjes, *op cit*, p. 67
3. *General Practitioner*, 2 May 1986
4. 'The problem of recurrent miscarriage', handout for women enquiring about immunology treatment at St Mary's Hospital
5. Stanway, *op cit*, p. 38
6. Huntingford, *op cit*, p. 61

5.
OLD WIVES' TALES?

Medlar: The fruit is Saturn's. It stays women's longings. A plaster made of the fruit dried before they are rotten, and other convenient things, and applied to the reins of the back, stops miscarriage in pregnant women.

CULPEPPER'S *Herbal*

Pregnancy, because it is so significant, so mysterious, and so little under our control, inspires superstitious beliefs: 'You shouldn't hang curtains when you're pregnant, or the cord will get wrapped round the baby's neck'; 'If you see a hare when you're pregnant, your baby will have a hare lip'; 'If you see a handicapped child when you're pregnant, you'll have one yourself.' Beliefs like these were quite widespread in our parents' or grand-parents' generation, but now we would probably dismiss them as 'old wives' tales'.

There are a lot of beliefs about what causes miscarriage that might seem to belong in the same category. Beliefs that miscarriage can be caused by falling downstairs, by having a distressing experience, by overdoing things, by worrying, or by making love. Most books directed at pregnant women nowadays will tell you that these things cannot cause miscarriage. Yet many women, knowing this, still wonder whether factors like over-exertion, or sexual intercourse, or a sudden shock, had something to do with their miscarriage.

In this chapter, I want to look at some further factors in miscarriage. This mixed bag of possibilities will include some of the 'old wives' tales'.

EXERCISE

It used to be widely believed that vigorous exercise and

generally 'overdoing it' made a woman more likely to miscarry. Nowadays such ideas have fallen out of favour. Advice to take things easy in pregnancy seems to evoke a past era of smelling salts and fainting fits and frail femininity. Pregnant women now prefer not to make concessions to what used to be called their 'condition', sometimes even cycling or swimming virtually up to the birth. Anecdotes about pregnant sportswomen winning Olympic medals seem to justify this approach to pregnancy.

For most women this approach does not pose any risk, but occasionally physical exertion can be risky. Vigorous exercise raises body heat and may divert blood away from the uterus. Both these processes might endanger the fetus. An expert on the subject writes, 'Direct human evidence that strenuous activity impairs blood flow to the uterus and has a deleterious effect on the fetus is not available but a great many straws are blowing in that direction.'[1]

There is a large margin of safety. Even when the mother's body is working vigorously, the blood flow to the uterus will usually be adequate. However a sudden severe bout of exercise — hill climbing, for instance — could endanger the fetus, and so could less vigorous activity, if the fetus is, for some reason, already at risk.

In the past, many doctors recommended that women who had suffered recurrent miscarriages should give up exercise entirely and stay in bed. Bedrest has a number of disadvantages. It's difficult for the woman to fit in with the rest of her life and her other commitments. It puts her at risk of other health problems, such as deep vein thrombosis. It forces her to focus on the pregnancy and her fears about it, to the exclusion of anything else. Many doctors now doubt whether bedrest ever has any value.

It is worth noting that a Swedish team who achieved impressive results with women who had suffered recurrent miscarriage did recommend two weeks' bedrest around the time that the woman had miscarried in the previous pregnancy. However their success is usually attributed to the 'optimal psychological support' they offered their patients, rather than the advice they gave.

INTERNAL/VAGINAL EXAMINATIONS

A number of women have described starting to miscarry a few hours after a vaginal examination in early pregnancy.

Sally said, 'At eleven weeks I went to hospital for my first book-in appointment. The doctor gave me a rather rough internal examination which, although it worried me a little, I thought must have been routine. The following day I started to bleed.' Sadly, Sally did lose her baby.

Sally's suspicions can easily be explained away. As you hunt around for ways to make sense of a miscarriage, you may latch on to anything that happened just before you started to bleed. If you had an internal examination the day before, you might blame the miscarriage on that, but this could simply be coincidence. There is no way of proving that the miscarriage was caused by the internal examination.

It is in fact unlikely that miscarriages can be caused by internal examinations, but it is not impossible. Later in pregnancy, stimulation of the cervix can cause prostaglandins to be released, and prostaglandins are involved in the process by which labour starts. It is presumably possible that stimulation of the cervix could occasionally also trigger off a miscarriage.

Since ultrasound became available, many obstetricians have stopped doing vaginal examinations in early pregnancy. It is a change that women welcome. Most women hate internals — they are intensely embarrassing, because of the sexual meanings of the examination, and they are often physically uncomfortable. We would tolerate the discomfort and the embarrassment if the examination was likely to give crucial information that would affect our treatment in a significant way, but this is unlikely. Even if there is only the slightest suspicion that an internal examination could trigger a miscarriage in an unstable pregnancy, it is plainly best avoided.

Remember, if you do not want an internal examination, you do not have to have one. Claire miscarried after a 'gentle' internal at 10 weeks. In her next pregnancy she started to spot at 8 weeks. 'At 11 weeks I refused an internal examination — having had a scan at 6½ weeks I felt an internal was unnecessary. My consultant was not too pleased, in fact he was downright rude in my opinion, so I took a deep breath and asked to change consultants!'

SEX

'With both my miscarriages,' Myra said, 'we'd made love the night before I started to bleed. No-one can convince me that having sex didn't have something to do with it. In my next pregnancy, we didn't have sex at all for the first three months. I bled a little at 8 weeks, but it stopped, and after that everything was fine.'

Sexual activity is frequently blamed for miscarriage. Men as well as women, searching for reasons for the miscarriage, may recall that they made love a day or two before it happened and wonder if that was the cause. Is this just a manifestation of that familiar association between sex and guilt? Or could they sometimes be right?

No-one knows for sure, but it is known that sexual activity can cause a woman who is already at term to go into labour. A woman's orgasm causes the womb to contract, and the sex researchers Masters and Johnson found that these contractions could trigger labour. Also, a man's semen contains protaglandins, substances that cause the cervix to dilate at the start of labour. Most of the time, these two effects of sexual intercourse probably only trigger labour in women who are just about ready to give birth anyway, but little is known about the complex mechanism by which labour starts. In the present state of knowledge, there is no known reason why these effects might not occasionally start the cervix dilating before the baby was ready.

For these reasons, in the next pregnancy after a miscarriage you will probably be advised not to make love at all for the first 14 weeks. Alternatively you might be advised to avoid making love at the times when your period would be due, at 8 and 12 weeks, as these seem to be the times when the risks of miscarriage are highest. For some women, though, making a conscious choice does not entirely solve the problem. Jane and her partner had decided to avoid sex for the first 14 weeks, but as Jane recalled, 'I stayed up late reading a rather randy novel, and I had an orgasm when I was asleep. I got in a real state about it. After that I took a gardening book to bed with me!'

PHYSICAL INJURY

If folk wisdom is to be believed, falling down the stairs is one of the most common causes of miscarriage. In the real world, however, it is very unlikely that you will miscarry as a result of falling over, even if you hurt yourself quite badly.

In the first trimester, the womb is well-protected by the pelvic bones. Later, as it grows, the fetus does become more vulnerable, but injury remains a very unusual cause of miscarriage. There have, however, been reports of women suffering miscarriage after suffering severe injury, for instance in road traffic accidents. Women who get beaten up by their husbands sometimes suffer miscarriages following these assaults. Being beaten up very badly might cause some separation of the placenta from the wall of the uterus, leading to miscarriage.

TWINS

The use of ultrasound scanning in early pregnancy has revealed some intriguing facts about twin conceptions. It seems that there are more twins in early pregnancy than would be expected from their frequency at birth.

Sometimes there are two amniotic sacs, but only one contains an embryo. In these cases, there are two possible outcomes. Either both sacs will be miscarried, or else just the empty sac will be miscarried, in which case the baby may be carried to term. When two embryos were conceived, it is possible for just one to die and be miscarried, and for the pregnancy to continue with a single embryo. This accounts for those unusual cases where a woman appears to have miscarried one baby, but remains pregnant.

It is not only early in pregnancy that miscarriage is more common in twin pregnancies. Late miscarriages caused by cervical incompetence are more common too, perhaps because there is more strain on the cervix. The miscarriage risk goes up still more with triplets and other multiple pregnancies.

AGE

Women over 35 are more likely than younger women to miscarry. This is probably because some sorts of chromosomal abnormalities become more common with age. The abnormalities in question are the 'trisomies', in which the chromosomes are grouped not in pairs, as they should be, but in threes. Down's Syndrome is an example of a trisomy. When 38-year-old women are given amniocentesis, less than 1 in 100 of their babies are shown to have Down's Syndrome. Among 45-year-old women, the proportion is 1 in 20. The proportion at both ages is obviously much higher earlier in pregnancy, as 9 out of 10 fetuses with Down's Syndrome will have been miscarried before 16 weeks.

If you do miscarry in your late thirties, it may take you longer to get pregnant again, as fertility declines somewhat after 35. It may take the average woman over 35 nearly twice as long to conceive as a woman in the 15 to 24 age group.[2] Some, but not all, of this decline is accounted for by the fact that couples who have been together for a number of years may make love less often.

Nowadays women are having babies later in life. As new kinds of life patterns for women emerge, many women are choosing to pursue their careers through their twenties and early thirties, before they think about getting pregnant. If you first try to conceive when you are 35, take a year to manage it, and then miscarry, you may have a despairing sense that you have simply left it too late. Many women feel a sense of panic as they read the statistics about miscarriage and Down's Syndrome and declining fertility. That nasty term 'elderly primagravida' does nothing to boost the confidence of women who fear that time is running out. Monica summed up these feelings. 'Next month I shall be 35 years old, so I must get over this terrible longing I have for another baby. I try to put it out of my mind during the day, but at night I often dream I am pregnant, or nursing my own child in my arms.'

It is easy to get a distorted impression of the risks and difficulties of trying to have a baby in your thirties. The risks of abnormality do increase after 35, but it is only one kind of abnormality — Down's Syndrome — that increases markedly, and that can be detected by amniocentesis. Fertility does decline after 35, but pregnancy is still possible. At 34, Monica has plenty of child-bearing years ahead of her. There are many women who even after a series of miscarriages, or years of infertility with occasional miscarriages, finally achieve their ambition in their late thirties or early forties and give birth to healthy babies.

DIET

There is a long tradition that links the mother's diet with the health of the baby in the womb. For instance, a seventeenth-century manual for midwives says, 'It is better for women with child to eat too much than too little, lest the child should want nourishment.'[3]

This old wisdom, however, was forgotten when male obstetricians took over the care of pregnant women from female midwives. At the end of the eighteenth century, doctors began to advocate restrictive diets during pregnancy. The theory was that if the mother's weight gain was restricted, the birth would be easier because the baby would be smaller. In our own century, the same practice has had a different justification. Women have been put on restrictive diets in an attempt to protect them from toxaemia, although research has shown that this dangerous illness of late pregnancy can be avoided by eating a high calorie, high protein diet. Vestiges of this approach are still apparent in the advice given in many ante-natal clinics. Women are still told off for gaining 'too much' weight in pregnancy.

Doctors who told pregnant women to restrict their weight gain believed that the baby was a parasite. The baby, it was thought, would not be harmed if the mother's diet was poor. It would get what it needed from the mother's system regardless of what she ate. However the baby is no parasite. If the mother is poorly nourished, so will the baby be. Evidence is accumulating that what the mother eats matters a great deal, and that poor diet may play a role in some miscarriages. Let's look at some of the evidence.

Firstly, there is evidence from animal experiments. When animals are deliberately fed diets low in vitamins[4] or low in trace elements[5] (such as zinc and iron), there is an increased miscarriage rate and an increased rate of congenital abnormalities. There are pitfalls in applying conclusions from animal experiments to humans, but these results do point to the importance of adequate nutrition in reproduction.

Secondly, there is evidence that giving women certain supplements for a month before and during the early weeks of pregnancy dramatically reduces the risk that their babies will be born with certain defects. Women who already have a spina bifida baby, and therefore had a 1 in 20 chance of having another, had a much better chance of having a healthy baby if they were given either a supplement of folic acid plus vitamins[6] or a supplement of folic acid alone[7] for at least a month before conception and for the early weeks of pregnancy. In one study, 9 per cent of the women not taking folic acid had another spina bifida baby, but all the women taking folic acid had normal babies. Folic acid is found in fresh green leafy vegetables, so women who eat few fresh vegetables will probably be deficient in this nutrient. There is also evidence that vitamin supplementation before and after conception may prevent cleft palate.

Thirdly, there is evidence that people who are severely undernourished have more miscarriages, as well as other reproductive problems. Such evidence, of course, cannot be acquired experimentally, but studies of people who suffered malnutrition during the Second World War have shown greatly increased miscarriage rates. From August 1940 to December 1942, Leningrad was under seige by the Nazis, and during this time no food could be shipped into the city. Many women stopped menstruating and only a few conceived. Among those who did conceive, there was a great increase in the rates of miscarriage, stillbirth, infant mortality and low birth weight.[8]

If poor diet means more reproductive problems then this is one way of understanding the links between poverty and miscarriage, for, as we shall see, women on low incomes suffer more miscarriages than other women. There is at least one study linking the incidence of spina bifida births with deprivation that implies that poor diet may be the link. Belfast has the highest rate of spina bifida births in the developed world. It also has a lower consumption of fresh fruit and fresh non-root vegetables per head than other parts of the UK. The rate of spina bifida births is highest specifically in the most deprived parts of the city. Families in these areas eat few fresh fruit or vegetables, both because of the expense and because of the difficulty of getting to shops that sell them.[9] A deficiency in folic acid in the women's diet, then, may be one link between deprivation and spina bifida in this particular instance. And it may also explain many miscarriages, as in Belfast 36 per cent of miscarried fetuses have neural tube defects such as spina bifida.

Fourthly, there is evidence that a good diet may protect you from the worst effects of certain poisons. For instance, a high intake of friendly minerals like calcium will prevent much lead being absorbed into your body. Animal experiments supply supporting evidence for the idea that diet has a protective effect. For instance, when thalidomide was given to pregnant rats, the well-nourished rats had undamaged babies, but the offspring of the poorly nourished rats had deformities similar to those found in humans exposed to the drug while in the womb.[10]

There is then a significant body of evidence suggesting that diet is important for a healthy pregnancy, but a doctor who sees you after a miscarriage is very unlikely to ask what you have been eating. Doctors are given little or no training in nutrition. The expert on diet is peripheral to the drama of modern obstetrics, with the nutritionist being given only a minor walk-on part in most ante-natal clinics. For most doctors, nutrition is simply not part of their frame of reference. A recent and otherwise comprehensive textbook for doctors — Huisjes' *Spontaneous Abortion* — makes no mention of nutrition.

POVERTY AS A REPRODUCTIVE HAZARD

Miscarriage — like pre-term labour, stillbirth, birth defects and perinatal mortality — is much more common among women on low incomes. We have discussed some of the individual factors that may increase the risk of miscarriage, but for women and men on low incomes a number of these risk factors may come together.

Take a woman living on a low income in poor housing. It is probable that her diet will be inadequate, as it takes great energy and ingenuity to eat well on a low income. Both she and her husband are more likely than middle-class people to work with dangerous chemicals or other hazards. As her flat is damp, she is more likely to suffer illness during pregnancy. Certain illnesses, such as respiratory tract infections, are ten times more common among people living in such conditions.[11] Poor diet, toxic hazards and illness — such factors, of course, by no means explain all miscarriages, but they do mean the scales are weighted against the woman on a low income, even before she conceives.

The medical model of illness means that the vital importance of such factors in miscarriage, or any other medical problem, may be overlooked. The woman is seen in hospital or in surgery. The emphasis is on her body not her circumstances. Most doctors show little interest in her exposure to toxic hazards or whether she can afford to eat properly.

It is a common misconception that our improved health as compared with, for instance, our Victorian ancestors, is due to the progress of medical science. In fact, cleaner water, better housing, better food and better living conditions generally have done much more to improve people's health than drugs or sophisticated surgical techniques.

In the case of any individual woman, her living conditions and diet may have nothing to do with her miscarriages, but it does seem likely that any improvements in the living conditions of the least privileged people in our society would have among its many effects on the nation's health a drop in the miscarriage rate.

Here are some thought-provoking statistics: 'In 19th century Europe, the infant mortality rate in the tenements was around 200 deaths per 1,000 babies. In the royal families at the same time it was about 12 deaths per 1,000 babies. That is almost as low as the most medically advanced country today with the most sophisticated of drugs available. Yet it was before any significant pharmaceutical breakthrough had occurred.'[12]

STRESS

Hippocrates, in the fifth century BC, warned pregnant women to avoid unnecessary psychic stress. His warning is still very much with us. The belief that stress is damaging in pregnancy often lies behind the kind of advice that friends and doctors give to pregnant women and women who have miscarried. It is apparent too in women's own beliefs about why they miscarried. Let's look at three different kinds of stress and ask whether they can cause miscarriage.

First, there is the most dramatic kind of stress — a sudden shock, such as a bereavement, or being mugged, or being made homeless. Pamela who lost her baby at 21 weeks, said, 'The house was burgled two weeks before I lost the baby. The place was ransacked. I was terribly upset, I let it get me down, which I shouldn't have, I suppose. Now I wonder whether that could have caused the miscarriage.'

There is some animal evidence which suggests that a sudden severe stress can trigger miscarriage. It is not known whether this happens in humans too, but it is recognized that a woman's menstrual cycle may be affected by shock. She may stop ovulating, or her periods may stop altogether, because her state of mind interferes with the working of the pituitary gland, which makes some of the hormones involved in female cycles. If shock can affect a woman's hormone levels in this way, then shock might in theory occasionally lead to miscarriage. However this remains guesswork. If it does happen at all, shock remains a very unlikely cause of miscarriage.

Secondly, there is the idea that work outside the home is a stress for women. The woman who has had a miscarriage may be advised by friends, relatives or doctors to give up work in her next pregnancy. Implicit in this advice is the notion that her work might have been responsible for her miscarriage. There is no scientific basis for this theory. Unless you are exposed to toxic hazards or radiation at work there is absolutely no reason to consider that your work might have played a part in your miscarriage.[13]

What then are the origins of this advice, so commonly given? In our society, outside employment for women is opposed to motherhood — the 'good mother' stays at home. Working mothers have been blamed for all manner of social problems from football hooliganism to drug addiction. I wonder if advice to pregnant women to give up work is rooted in this opposition between work and motherhood. Perhaps it is a variant of 'good mothers stay at home' — the belief that you can only care properly for your children, even when they are still in the womb, by giving up work and taking on the feminine role of home-maker.

In fact, being at home is not necessarily easier — physically or emotionally — than being engaged in outside work. Housework is more physically strenuous than, for instance, sitting at an office desk, and looking after small children is more exhausting than almost any other form of work. However, it is not often suggested that women should give up these forms of work in pregnancy. Emotionally, too, being at home can be difficult. A large-scale study of the mental health of women identified the lack of outside employment as a major stress for women.[14] Women at home are more likely to suffer from depression, anxiety symptoms, phobias and other psychological ills than women with outside employment.

If you are wondering whether to give up work to give your next pregnancy the best possible chance, think hard and long before you take that step. You might be less tired and more content if you paid for extra childcare and help with the housework, and stayed on at work.

Thirdly, there is the idea that 'worry' causes miscarriage. Some doctors have suggested that women who suffer recurrent miscarriages get in such an anxious state because they have miscarried in the past that this actually makes another miscarriage more likely.

There are plenty of hints that what goes on in our heads does affect our fertility, but the link between thinking and reproduction is subtle and mysterious. For instance, it often seems to happen that a couple who have been infertile for years and have applied to adopt a child, suddenly conceive when their names come to the top of the list of prospective adoptive parents. It is simplistic to suggest that they become fertile because they are worrying less, for in some ways this must be a time of increased worry and stress for them. Yet for some couples, this situation seems to bring about a shift in their thinking and feeling that makes it possible for them to conceive.

There is one way you can bring about such a shift in yourself as you approach your next pregnancy and that is to find a doctor whom you can trust and who makes you feel confident and cared for. Many women attribute their successes to this and there is some evidence that supports this belief.

Studies have shown that any new treatment has a high success rate with women who have suffered recurrent miscarriage. If new treatment — whatever it is — works well for a lot of women, it is likely that it is something other than the treatment itself that matters. As you would expect from that result, when women are offered a placebo — a dummy treatment — there is also a high success rate. In other words, what the woman thinks about her treatment is very important. She may still worry — in fact, if she is given a new treatment which involves travel, inconvenience, expense and perhaps unpleasant side-effects, she will be even more preoccupied with her pregnancy and the possibility of miscarriage than if she was not being treated. However two things have changed for the better — she now feels hope as well as anxiety, and she has a relationship with a doctor whom she feels is responding to her need.

The importance of the relationship with the doctor, and what he or she offers apart from treatment, is confirmed by a study from Sweden.[15] This study found that 'optimal psychological support' of women with a history of recent miscarriage resulted in a high success rate. Nearly 200 women who had suffered recurrent miscarriage were screened for physical problems. Abnormalities were found in about half of them and these women were treated. Of the women in this group, 80 per cent who subsequently conceived carried their pregnancies to term. The other group of women, in whom no abnormalities were found, were seen every week for a medical examination, and they were offered 'optimal psychological support'. Apart from this care and support they were given no treatment, although they were given advice which included resting, no sex, and staying in bed for 2 weeks at the stage of pregnancy at which they had last miscarried. Of these women 86 per cent carried their pregnancies to term.

Healers in every culture and age have recognized that their relationship with their patients is a vital dimension of healing. In recent years in Western medicine, this truth has been forgotten. Thinking about medicine has been restricted by a narrow definition of 'science', or so you would imagine from the way doctors write, or the way medical students are educated, although even in the most unpromising settings there have always been some doctors who recognized the roles of faith, hope and love in their work. Fortunately attitudes are changing. In the treatment of women who have suffered recurrent miscarriage there is an increasing awareness of the importance of thoughts and feelings, although the physical mechanism that translates a woman's trust and optimism into a successful pregnancy is still not understood.

It is appropriate to end this section that deals with the causes of miscarriage on a note of mystery and uncertainty. For most of us, as we try to make sense of our miscarriages, there are lots of unanswered questions. And that is not only true on the individual level. Many of our more general questions, too, may receive only speculative and incomplete answers. Given the present state of knowledge about miscarriage, our hunger for information can at best be only partially satisfied.

SOURCES

Geoffrey Chamberlain (ed) *Pregnant Women At Work*, The Royal Society of Medicine and the Macmillan Press Ltd, London, 1984

Barbara Luke, *Maternal Nutrition*, Little, Brown and Co., Boston, 1979

Barbara Pickard, *Eating Well For A Healthy Pregnancy*, Sheldon, London, 1984

Gail Sforza Brewer with Tom Brewer, *What Every Pregnant Woman Should Know*, Penguin, Harmondsworth, 1985

REFERENCES

1. F.E. Hytten, 'The effect of work on placental function and fetal growth,' in Chamberlain, *op cit*, p. 22
2. A.H. DeCherney and G.S. Berkowitz, 'Female fecundity and age', *New England Journal of Medicine*, vol. 306, no., 7. 8 February 1982, p. 424
3. N. Culpepper, *A Directory For Midwives*, quoted in Luke, *op cit*
4. I.W. Jennings, 'Hormones and vitamins in pre-natal life,' in *Vitamins In Endocrine Metabolism*, Heinemann, London, 1970, pp. 126-42
5. E.J. Underwood, *Trace Elements In Human And Animal Nutrition*, New Academic Press, New York and London, 1977
6. Smithells *et al*, 'Apparent prevention of neural tube defects by peri-conceptional vitamin supplementation', *Archives of Disease in Childhood*, 56, 1981, pp. 911-18
7. Lawrence *et al*, 'Double-blind randomised controlled trial of folate treatment before conception to prevent recurrence of neural-tube defects', *British Medical Journal*, vol. 282, 1981, pp. 1509-11
8. Brewer, *op cit*
9. M. Hyndeman of Northern Visions Ltd, personal communication
10. Fratta *et al*, 'Teratogenic effects of thalidomide in rabbits, rats, hamsters and mice', *Toxicology and Applied Pharmacology* vol. 7, 1965, pp. 268-86
11. *The Guardian*, 15 December 1986
12. *The New Internationalist*, November 1968, p. 17, quoting statistics from *The State of The World's Children*, 1986
13. Peters *et al*, 'The effects of work in pregnancy: short and long-term associations' in Chamberlain, *op cit*, p. 87
14. George Brown and Tirril Harris, *Social Origins of Depression*, Tavistock, London, 1978
15. B. Stray-Pedersen and S. Stray-Pedersen, 'Etiologic factors and subsequent reproductive performance in 195 couples with a prior history of habitual abortion', *American Journal of Obstetrics and Gynaecology*, vol. 148, no. 2, 15 January 1984, p. 140

6.
WOMEN'S FEELINGS

Lullay, lullay, my lityl chyld,
Slepe and be now styll.
ANON (fifteenth century)

I used to think my first miscarriage hadn't touched me. I have a picture of myself sitting in the car in the hospital car park, ready to go home. I can remember every detail of that landscape of concrete and tarmac and grey sky, but the picture is somehow unreal, almost as though it was a detail from somebody else's life. I remember thinking to myself, 'How odd, I don't feel upset, in fact I don't feel anything at all.' Although the baby had been planned and wanted, that miscarriage seemed to mean nothing to me. I simply blotted it out of my mind.

It is only since I started writing this book that I have started to think back to that experience and my lack of reaction, and to wonder what was going on. I have recalled that the year that followed the miscarriage was one of the unhappiest in my life. Time and again I picked up projects, then abandoned them. Nothing seemed worthwhile, nothing could be brought to completion. It was as though, rather than grieving, I was acting out the theme of miscarriage in everything I did. A year after the miscarriage, my first marriage ended. I have come to realize that the miscarriage in fact had a profound effect on me, an effect that I had always denied.

For me, the distress of miscarriage was hidden or postponed. For another woman the pain is vivid and immediate. Each woman's response is unique, woven from our individual situations and personalities. Yet the varying textures of our stories are shot through with threads of similar colours, the themes that recur.

SADNESS

Emma lost her baby at 20 weeks.

> When I arrived home from hospital, I was fine until I went
> into our back bedroom which we had been in the process of
> converting into a nursery. My husband had removed the
> baby equipment we had accumulated and the room was bare
> and abandoned. I think it was then that I realized what had
> happened to us. I began to experience the first sharp
> agonizing and bitter grief and shock of miscarriage. This grief
> seems unbearable and unending, it seems to give rise to an
> almost physical internal pain.

The loss of a child at any age is the most distressing and long-
lasting of all griefs. No wonder there is such pain in miscarriage,
for the woman who experiences it as the loss of a child.

Sally lost her baby at 11 weeks — 'I cried constantly, broke
down in public on two separate occasions, could think and talk
of nothing else. Paul came home from work every day to find me
lying on the bed asking again and again why my baby had died.'
Crying is the usual and natural expression of grief. However
strong and independent she is, the woman who grieves after
miscarriage will find herself constantly weeping, or struggling to
keep back the tears. She may worry that the crying will never
stop.

Grief also means preoccupation. People who have lost
someone close to them are preoccupied with thoughts of the lost
person, and with the days and hours that led up to the death.
Freud called this 'grief work', and saw it as a necessary part of
mourning. So, like Sally, the woman who has miscarried keeps
asking why it had to happen and whether it could have been
different. She wants others to listen as she re-tells her story,
though she may worry that her partner and her friends will lose
patience with all these repetitions. It is as though she has to
make sense of the miscarriage by reliving it again and again.
While she is in this state of preoccupation, life seems to lose its
meaning, and things that once gave her pleasure seem pointless.

An animal whose mate has died will spend days seeking for
it, wearing itself out in the search. The anxiety and restlessness
that bereaved people feel has its roots in this urge to search for
the lost person. There are vestiges of this searching impulse in
women's reactions after miscarriage. As Kathleen expressed it,
'I used to wonder where my baby was. I used to think about this
little lost soul just wandering around, looking for a new home.'
Sometimes the searching impulse has expression in our dreams.

A woman who has miscarried is said to have 'lost her baby'. In dreams this happens literally, you suddenly remember that you have had a baby and that you have left it behind in an egg box in the supermarket, or that you have forgotten to feed it and carelessly left it lying around. You look everywhere for it but the lost baby is not to be found.

Grief after miscarriage lasts a long time. Months later, just when you feel you are coping again, you are given a baby to cuddle, or a friend announces she is pregnant, and the sadness surges back. It has a way of returning, too, on anniversaries, or at a time of year that you associate with the lost pregnancy. Jennifer said, 'When the forsythia started to flower, I thought — the forsythia was flowering last year when I had the miscarriage.'

EMPTINESS

Pamela McDonald remembers, 'There was this feeling that something was missing, that I had been interrupted in the middle of doing something, a feeling of emptiness as though I had mislaid something, but of not being quite sure what exactly it was.'[1]

Bereaved people and those who are depressed say they feel 'empty'. Just as 'fulfilment' means happiness and a sense of purpose, so being 'empty inside' suggests a state of sadness or despair. There is a very specific sense in which we are 'empty' after miscarriage.

In pregnancy, a woman is full — her body is literally full, containing and nurturing the baby, and her mind is full, too, full of plans and worries and questions. Will it be a boy or a girl? When shall I give up work? Shall I have an epidural? Will the butterfly wallpaper look good in the nursery? How on earth will I cope? Even in sleep, pregnant women are working on the future. Dreams in pregnancy are unusually vivid. We dream about giving birth to strange creatures, or about being born ourselves — pushing through a revolving door, or being whirled down a dark tunnel. We dream about looking after babies. Myra recalls one of her dreams while pregnant: 'I dreamt about having to look after a wild horse in the cosmetics department of a large store. I knew the dream was about having the baby, and how unprepared I was. I only had perfumes and lipsticks, when what I needed was a bridle and reins.'

Then suddenly all that work of body and mind comes to an end. After miscarriage, the woman's womb is literally empty. 'I lost a lot of blood,' Sandra said. 'I told my husband then I knew I had lost the baby because I felt so "empty".' Some women can sense the physical emptiness, but many women know its emotional equivalent, the empty womb of the mind.

MAKING IT REAL

'Coming to terms with inevitable death,' wrote Gill, 'is something which is almost beyond us. When it happens to a person we love, have loved through that person's life perhaps, or throughout our own, we cling on to their personality, their possessions, our memories of them. But when it happens to an unborn baby, we have nothing on which to lean. The blank face of death meets us and mentally we shy away.'

The baby inside her feels very real at times to the pregnant woman. She plans for it, names it, worries about it, and wonders what it will be like. Once she can feel movement she may have a sense of its personality. She notices that it always starts wriggling just when she lies down to sleep, or that it jumps in response to high-pitched voices singing on the radio. Some women are convinced they know the sex of the babies inside them.

When pregnancy ends in miscarriage, these intuitions and guesses are all a woman is left with. There are no drawers stuffed with photographs, no pictures even in the mind. To draw the form of a miscarried baby in memory, wrote one poet, is 'to sketch the shape of the rain'. Pregnancy is the most physically intimate of all relationships, yet in no other relationship is so little known about the other person. How can a woman grieve for someone about whom she knows so little? As Lorna expressed it, 'It doesn't matter at what stage a baby vanished from your body and your life, it's hard to come to terms with the silence which surrounds a baby who is not full-term.'

Some women see their babies. Diana did. 'I went to the loo and discovered a little bleeding. I wiped myself only to discover my baby, tiny but complete and incredibly beautiful, was in my hand. It was the most shocking thing that has ever happened to me. I was deeply distressed.' In the long term this disturbing experience can be a source of strength. It supplies what is missing for the woman who miscarries, an image on which she can focus her sense of loss. It is no longer only 'the blank face of death' that she sees in her mind's eye. She knows for whom she is grieving.

It is because of the need to 'make it real' that women want to know all that can be known about their lost babies. Often this takes the form of an urgent curiosity about the baby's sex. Our gender is a fundamental part of our identity. 'Is it a boy or a girl?' is the second question we ask when a baby is born, after

'Is it all right?' If you know your baby's sex, you can talk about the baby as a person, no longer 'it' but 'him' or 'her'.

Sue had a late miscarriage, at 23 weeks. She knew her baby was a girl, but craved to know more. 'Although sympathetic, the staff didn't ask me if I wanted to see or hold my baby. In fact I asked to see her but unfortunately didn't hold her. My GP couldn't understand why I wanted to find out such minor details as her weight and length and if a photo had been taken, and I was told to stop crucifying myself, especially when I mentioned my desire to know what had happened to her body.'

It may be very distressing to think of the baby's body being disposed of without ceremony. Some women have preferred to bury the baby themselves, as Kate did. 'I remember being amazed at the doctor's suggestion that we would perhaps like to have a service held in church for our baby. In the event we did not feel that we wanted a public service for our child that had not shared in public life, and we buried the baby privately. When we buried it we placed it with a little toy that had been, by chance, near at hand throughout the hours of the miscarriage, and, from the baby's two sisters, daisies that they had picked for me because I wasn't well.'

Making up a small ritual can be one way to 'make it real'. Other women have written poems, or planted rose bushes in the garden. By doing these things, women can begin to come to terms with that silence that surrounds a baby who has miscarried.

THE FEAR OF OVER-REACTING

'I think that I have over-reacted,' Gita admitted, 'but I can't help it. I feel such a sense of loss.' It is not surprising that women worry about over-reacting. There are few signs that other women feel like them. Miscarriage, although such a common event, is scarcely ever mentioned in public.

In our newspapers and novels and plays, there are many images of suffering women — the abandoned wife, the rape victim, the lonely housewife — but on this significant source of suffering there is almost total silence. There are one or two discreet references in Victorian novels, an equally discreet miscarriage shrouded in symbolism at the end of D.H. Lawrence's *The Rainbow*, an account of a man's experience of miscarriage in Stan Barstow's *A Kind of Loving*. Just a handful of exceptions to the rule of silence. Yet surely miscarriage lends itself to literary or dramatic treatment? Like death, disaster or falling in love, or any of the other events on which a plot may hinge, miscarriage changes people and the way they relate to one another.

The silence is still more surprising when it comes to advice given to pregnant women. Ante-natal clinics usually have a plentiful supply of information leaflets, full of pictures of delectable babies in snow-white nappies, and glossy women in bright dungarees, and pages of advice with words like 'never' and 'always' in heavy type. They say little or nothing about the way one in six pregnancies end. *The Baby Book*, for instance, has three sentences on miscarriage in its 144 pages.[2] To read these leaflets you would think miscarriage was very rare. You would certainly never suspect that it stirs up such painful and powerful feelings.

Loneliness is an inevitable part of grief, but the loneliness of miscarriage is intensified by the way these feelings are denied, as Monica found. 'The feeling of being alone with this particular grief was the worst thing about my miscarriage. I felt no-one could possibly feel as I did and I felt I had to hold the grief to myself.'

If a woman does allow herself to grieve openly, others may not be so generous. Elaine is a psychiatric nurse and knew from her training that grief needs to be expressed: 'Amid the other women on the ward I would curl up in bed and cry my heart out. I overheard two women saying how silly I was for not keeping a stiff upper lip.'

Women in certain situations are particularly vulnerable to accusations that they are over-reacting. It is as though there are unspoken but cruel rules about who may grieve after miscarriage. A little sadness may be permissible in the married woman whose pregnancy was planned, and who has no children already. But grief is not acceptable in the unmarried woman, the woman without a partner, the woman who got pregnant by accident, or the woman who already has two or three children. Cathy recalled, 'The remark that upset me most was from the nurse pushing my trolley into the theatre. When I told her my partner and I weren't married yet, she said that it was probably best that I'd lost the baby, and perhaps we could try again once we were married. Both of us had desparately wanted that baby and had been devastated by what had happened.'

LOSS OF MOTHERHOOD

'Pregnancy is the only key to that exclusive club. The reading *Mother* and *Parents* magazines club, the ante-natal club, the shopping for a newborn club, the maternity clothes club, all these activities which are suddenly and viciously no longer mine to indulge in.'

When a woman has a miscarriage, she not only loses the baby. She also loses an image of herself as mother. She is, at least for a while, excluded from the club.

When you are pregnant with your first child, you are very much preoccupied with the image of yourself as mother. On the blank slate of the future, you draw pictures — yourself holding or feeding a baby, pushing a pram, showing the baby to your parents. You may view these pictures you create with delighted anticipation, or with doubtful anxiety, most likely with a mixture of the two. When you miscarry, the pictures have to be rubbed out. At least for the moment, the future has to be drawn in a different way. The images of yourself as a mother have to be shelved, along with the baby equipment and the maternity clothes. As Lynn put it, 'I eventually returned to work, and although this in itself was therapeutic, I would often find myself reflecting on what might have been and this at first was very distressing. I would think "I should be at home with my baby."'

Being excluded from the club is a shock. Since 1927, when Marie Stopes parked her birth control caravan outside Bethnal Green library at the start of her campaign to bring advice on contraception to all women, our thinking about pregnancy has changed in a radical way. Women who have used contraception for years are often quite unprepared for the difficulties they may encounter once they do decide to have babies.

As a child I was fascinated by a poster in the local library, showing Mum and Dad and two children, in cheerful primary colours, and underneath a slogan urging everyone to plan their families. I puzzled over this. My mother had told me most emphatically that you could not choose when to have children, yet the poster seemed to promise that you could. The contradiction of course is easily resolved. You cannot choose when to have children — you can only choose when not to have them.

The belief that if you throw away your pills, then pregnancy and a baby will rapidly follow, is reinforced by recent advances in reproductive technology. Babies can be conceived in test-tubes. It is even claimed that the technology is now available for men to bear children, an idea that I took to be a bizarre joke when I first came across it. This is the background against which pregnancy fails. A woman may be amazed to learn that, in spite of the glittering technology, little can be done to help her with such a common reproductive problem as miscarriage. In these days of effective contraception and 'test-tube babies', reproduction remains a risky, wasteful and fallible affair.

ANGER

'I wanted to raise my fists to the sky and rant and rage at the trick, and scream at being denied,' wrote Pamela McDonald in her account of her miscarriage.[3]

Anger is part of grieving. The anger that Pamela feels is shared by many women in their grief after miscarriage. Like Pamela, women are angry with fate, providence, God — whatever or whoever in their philosophy of life they hold ultimately responsible for what has happened.

A woman may also feel angry with her GP or with the hospital staff. As she goes back over the experience in her mind, trying to make sense of it, she feels that someone has been negligent or callous. Sadly, many women who miscarry get appalling treatment from doctors and hospitals (see Chapter 9). When this makes women angry, their rage can be the driving force that brings about change for the better. Many reforms in the treatment of women — for instance, changes in the way childbirth is managed — have been brought about by women's anger. Hopefully, women's anger about the way some women who miscarry are treated will also lead to changes.

Sometimes anger with doctors has different roots. Doctors are an obvious target for the rage that people feel at the loss of loved ones. It is not unknown for doctors to be punched by people when they have just told them of the sudden death of relatives. After miscarriage a woman's rage may be directed at the doctor who told her that her baby was dead, or who literally took her baby away by doing a D & C. As Frances put it, 'I swore never again to trust a doctor. I think I was looking for someone to blame, on to whom I could transfer my irrational feeling of guilt.'

We are angry with God, and with doctors, because we see both as having power over life and death. This anger then makes some kind of sense, but one of the most common and painful forms of anger after miscarriage is rather less rational.

When you have just had a miscarriage, your world is suddenly teeming with pregnant women, women with placid faces and confident smiles and massive bodies that do not let them down. Some of them are women who did not want children, or at least not as passionately as you, yet they get pregnant effortlessly. They do all the 'wrong' things in pregnancy, drink and smoke and live on chips, yet they have beautiful full-term babies. Val said, 'When I see other women with babies or pregnant, I feel I want to cry and say horrible things to them.' Judith talked about 'the urge to push shopping trolleys into the pregnant bulge of another woman'.

Women use strong words to describe these feelings — terrible, hateful, devastating. Where it is a sister or sister-in-law who is pregnant the feelings may be particularly intense. After her own miscarriage, Lydia learned that her sister-in-law was pregnant. 'I was absolutely devastated. I felt as if someone had inflicted upon me the most dreadful physical pain, and I hated her so much it was unbelievable. . . . I couldn't bring myself to talk to my husband about these terrible feelings, because I wanted to call his own sister all the most dreadful names, and I hated her so much.'

Sometimes a woman feels a very specific anger, directed only at women who have got pregnant since her miscarriage, or women who have just given birth to a third child when it was her third baby that miscarried. Joy said, 'Months later I would still have moments of bitterness — usually when I heard of someone who'd had a miscarriage, and had known what sex the baby was.' Sometimes the anger is directed at women who've chosen to have abortions. Liz described feelings of 'hate' for a woman she knew who had had an abortion. 'I began to feel so angry that many women have to go through the agonies of miscarriage with the loss of a much wanted baby while this person had aborted a viable pregnancy.'

Filling up with rage, resentment and bitterness towards women in her own family or among her circle of friends, a woman comes to feel she must be a very bad person. She starts avoiding people, finding herself unable to pick up the phone to talk to women she used to be fond of. She knows her anger is irrational, but it is deeply felt and hard to control. And it can blaze on for a long time, only slowly dying down, changing into what one woman called 'a kind of burnt-out bitterness'.

History provides a dramatic example of angry and violent feelings provoked in part by miscarriage. Thirty years ago Ruth Ellis was hanged for shooting dead her lover, David Blakely. A few days before she shot him, she had suffered a miscarriage. In her case the trauma of miscarriage was compounded by the fact that David Blakely's violence to her almost certainly caused the miscarriage — she had started to bleed shortly after he had beaten her up. Her defence counsel made no use whatever of the miscarriage in her defence at the trial.

GUILT

'I blame myself. I should have listened to myself — and not taken any of these medicines. No wonder my baby died. I can't forgive myself.'

Variations on that first phrase come again and again when women tell the stories of their miscarriages. 'I blame myself.' 'I can't forgive myself.' 'I feel so guilty.' We look back and remember something we did. I moved that dustbin, made love, didn't give up work, ate the wrong things, didn't go to bed when the bleeding started. ... Occasionally we blame ourselves for things which do put up the risks of miscarriage a bit — smoking and drinking, for instance. More often, we blame ourselves for something that could not possibly have had anything to do with the miscarriage.

Sometimes we put the blame not on our bodies but on our thoughts and feelings. A woman may believe that the cause of the miscarriage was a failure of love. She didn't love the baby enough, or she didn't express that love when the baby most needed it. Babies once born are dependent on our love for their survival. The kind of love they evoke in us is in part a response to their vulnerability. It is a love which has a huge component of protectiveness. The death of a baby inside your body can feel like a failure of that love. Michelle expressed it like this: 'I shall never forgive myself for throwing away my tiny baby. I tried so hard to save it, but I let it down. I failed my baby and myself and nothing can change that.'

A woman may come to believe that the pregnancy miscarried because she did not feel the 'right' kind of love for the baby. She is most likely to believe this if the pregnancy was not planned, and she was shocked and upset to find herself pregnant. Another woman may feel she did not act on her love at the right time or in the right way.

Ros lost her baby at 12 weeks. 'Had I been more conscious that I might lose the baby, would I have felt more for it during the three months I carried it, would I have put it first whenever my toddler wanted to be lifted up and carried? When I saw my dead baby I could not have loved it more than I did, but by then it was too late.'

Veronica lost her twins later in pregnancy. 'The first little girl was still-born, the second little girl was alive — she cried, they took her away, I never saw her — what happened to her? I was asked if I wanted to see her. I was scared. I knew she wouldn't survive and I said no — did I condemn her to death by refusing to look at her?'

I wonder if these ideas have their roots in moments when we feel powerful love for our children or our unborn babies. At such times we can feel almost omnipotent. Loving our children so intensely, we may believe that by our love we can protect them from bad things and keep them alive. It follows that we may come to believe that if we do not love them enough they will die.

But the world does not work like that, and the belief that it does is a terrible burden for any woman to carry.

I think there is another strand of meaning here too. There is also the theme of miscarriage as punishment. The miscarriage is seen as evidence of and punishment for our badness and our failures of love. A woman may believe that by having the wrong feelings or by doing something wrong in the past, she has brought the miscarriage on herself. This belief, of course, is not unique to miscarriage. Other disasters, too, may be seen as punishment for bad things we have done, but I think it is a particularly powerful strand in our thinking about reproduction.

When I started thinking about the theme of miscarriage as punishment, I was intrigued to notice that certain fairy stories and legends have similar themes. Bad actions lead to the loss of a child, or the loss of a child is the punishment for some transgression or failure. In Rapunzel, for instance, the man steals salad for his wife from the witch's garden. The witch catches him at it, but lets him take the salad, on condition that in return she will take any baby the couple may have. In Rumpelstiltskin, the mannikin turns straw into gold for the miller's daughter. She rewards him with her ring and her necklace, but when she has no more jewels to give, she has to promise that he can take her first-born child. In the Legend of King Arthur, Ygraine unknowingly commits adultery with Uther, who is magically disguised as her husband and Merlin takes Arthur, the child of their union, as soon as he is born. In each story there is a sin or failure — stealing the salad, adultery, not rewarding for services rendered — and the loss of a child is the price that must be paid. Such stories suggest that the theme of the loss of a child as punishment for wrong-doing is a persistent part of human thinking about reproduction. No wonder we believe it so readily.

Such beliefs are common among women who have chosen to have abortions in the past. Studies have shown that, except where repeated D & C's may cause cervical incompetence, induced abortion does not increase your chances of having a miscarriage in a subsequent pregnancy. Yet a woman may still agonize about whether a past abortion caused the miscarriage. The 'crime' might also be some other kind of difficulty in the past, for instance, a messy marriage breakup. Or it might be an attitude you have held. As Pamela said, only half-jokingly, 'Perhaps it's a punishment for all those years of looking down on women who just wanted babies.'

DOUBTS ABOUT YOUR BODY

After her second miscarriage, Chris said, 'I began to think there
was something wrong with me.' Myra echoed this feeling after
her first miscarriage. 'It was a kind of confirmation of what I'd
always suspected. My periods didn't start properly till I was 18.
I'd just always known there was something wrong — that I
wasn't a proper woman.' Vera, who had had several
miscarriages, admitted, 'By now I no longer felt like a woman. I
felt so lonely and incomplete a total failure.'

Our reproductive organs are hidden from us. We cannot
check up on them. We have no way of knowing whether
everything is as it should be inside us. Only with pregnancy is
the working of those organs put to the test — and when you
miscarry you feel that you have failed. A miscarriage stirs up
fears that something is wrong deep inside.

As we have seen, problems with the mother's physiology only
account for a very small proportion of miscarriages, but knowing
this only goes a little way to assuage those doubts about our
bodies after miscarriage. These doubts have deep roots, and go
back a long way.

Throughout history, until the ovum was first seen with the
development of the microscope in the early nineteenth century,
the role of the woman in reproduction was seriously
underestimated. Mainstream Christian thought, for instance,
maintained that the embryo took its material substance from
the woman but all its vital qualities, its form and movement,
from the man.[4] Yet, however small a role the woman at various
epochs was believed to play in the genesis of the baby, she
would still be blamed if something went wrong. Infertility would
be blamed on her, and so would the birth of babies of the wrong
sex. Henry VIII divorced Katharine of Aragon because she
failed to produce a male heir. We know more now — for
instance, we know that the baby's sex is determined by the
sperm — but the belief that the woman's body is to blame for
pregnancy failures still leads to distortions. For instance,
research into the causes of pregnancy problems focuses almost
entirely on the woman, and there is little recognition of the
importance of protecting men as well as women from toxic
hazards at work.

Occasionally, of course, the results of tests will seem to
confirm a woman's fears that something is wrong with her body.
She may be told, for instance, that she has an abnormally
shaped uterus, or hormone deficiency, or cervical incompetence.
Abnormal, deficient, incompetent — the words themselves do
nothing for her self-esteem.

If a problem is diagnosed, she may have mixed feelings. She may be grateful that there is something to work on and that treatment may be possible. Yet she still has to cope with the knowledge that there is something wrong. Debbie had a hysterosalpingogram (womb X-ray). Looking at the screen, she could see that she had a 'weird-looking womb'. She says, 'When I look back now at that bleak morning when the hysterosalpingogram was performed, it seems like a dream. I had wanted to have the X-ray, and yet afterwards, let down by the amount of discomfort I had experienced and angry with my body for being less than perfect, I wondered if ignorance hadn't been bliss.'

WANTING ANOTHER BABY

'For months on end I wouldn't go out alone in case I saw an unattended baby in a pram. I was sure I would steal it,' remembers Sheila.

After miscarriage it is very common to yearn for another baby. Women talk about being 'obsessed' or 'taken over' by this yearning. Or they say they 'crave' a baby — as you crave a drug to which you are addicted, or water in a dry dusty place. The intensity of the feeling may be shocking. Since the re-emergence of feminism in the late sixties, many of us have learnt not to see ourselves solely in terms of our potential for having children. Feminist writers have focused on the grim side of motherhood, the hard work, boredom and isolation, and sometimes in opposing these things they have appeared to oppose the bearing and rearing of children too. Some feminist writers of fantasy have even conjured up Utopias in which biological motherhood no longer exists — like Marge Piercy's *Woman on the Edge of Time* in which babies develop in and are born from test-tubes. The stress on the grim side of motherhood was perhaps necessary, in a society that viewed motherhood as the only, or the most important, thing that women could do. Yet it leaves some women quite unprepared for the passions that pregnancy and miscarriage stir up. Pamela said, 'When it all went wrong, I thought, I've left it too late, I've thrown away all my chances. It made me review all my adult life — contraceptives I've used, all those years on the pill. Was there any point? Was it all worth it? I'm only a social worker, after all, I'm not Prime Minister or anything.'

Wanting another baby so much can also cause difficulties with a woman's partner, especially if the original pregnancy was not part of the couple's plans. The story may go like this. A woman gets pregnant by accident. At first she is shocked and upset, but gradually she comes to accept and even welcome the idea of having a baby. Then, just when she has got used to the idea, she miscarries. Her immediate response is to want to get pregnant again. The man on the other hand is relieved that the pregnancy has ended. He simply cannot understand her yearning for a baby.

Sometimes the longing for another baby will be tinged with fear. What if you do get pregnant, but it all goes wrong again? Looking back to this period in her life, Sophie acknowledges her mixed feelings. 'We didn't take precautions, but when we did make love we banked on withdrawal. Simply because in one way we wanted a baby, yet in another way we didn't.'

THE NEED TO BREAK THE TABOO

Anna spoke for many women when she asked, 'Why hadn't I known about miscarriage before it actually happened to me? Why had it never been mentioned on the women's programmes, or in the magazines or newspapers? There was always plenty about contraception, planned abortion, menopause and even sterilization, but why not about miscarriage? Weren't women suffering them every day? I scoured bookshops and magazines hoping to read something of women who had suffered like me, to glean some comfort from their experiences and how they survived them, but there was this dreadful silence on the subject.' Women's experiences of miscarriage cannot be understood without considering that 'dreadful silence' that Anna describes.

Miscarriage means the death of a baby. And some of those responses to miscarriage are part of something wider — responses to loss, death and bereavement. It is natural to fear death, to want to avoid thinking about death, and to feel uncomfortable in the company of people who have been bereaved. Our own society is not unique in this. Some cultures have customs that legitimize these reactions — for instance, recently widowed women may be shunned — but it does seem likely that changes over the past fifty years have made dying and bereavement harder to cope with. Most people die in hospital away from familiar surroundings and loved relatives. Few adults have ever seen a dead body. Traditional customs that helped people to express their grief — wearing black clothes for instance — have largely been abandoned. There is a paradox here — death is at once familiar and strange. Death is constantly before us on our television screens, yet the dead and dying are shut away from our day-to-day lives, and the expression of grief is taboo.

In many societies other than our own, the inner desolation of grief is given outward expression in elaborate rituals. And in most, death is part of the texture of everyday life. It is possible that in such a society, a woman who loses a baby, at whatever stage of pregnancy, will meet with less denial and more understanding and will find it easier to grieve. Occasionally anthropologists have described societies in which mourning rituals are extended to the miscarried baby. The Siriono Indian people, for instance, apparently mourn a miscarriage for three days, with the same rites used for any person who has died.[5] The custom implies a very different attitude to death and in particular to miscarriage. In our own society, a woman who wants a funeral for her miscarried baby may be seen as eccentric or morbid.

However the death taboo is only a partial explanation of those walls of silence that surround miscarriage. The denial of death in our culture does not explain why the particular loss of miscarriage is singled out for such conscientious avoidance. In order to understand more fully, we need to look elsewhere, to the menstrual taboo.

Menstrual blood is seen as unclean, dangerous and polluting in many cultures. It is one of the oldest and most widespread taboos, in fact the very word taboo is said to originate from the Polynesian word for menstruation, 'tupua'. The Roman philosopher Pliny in his 'Natural History' tells us that menstrual blood 'turns new wine sour, crops touched by it become barren, grafts die, seed in gardens are dried up, the fruit of trees falls off, the edge of steel and the gleam of ivory are dulled, hives of bees die.'[6]

In many societies, the behaviour of menstruating women has been controlled by strict rules. They may not be allowed to cook or to touch cooking pots. They may have to spend the days when they are menstruating away from their village in menstrual huts. There have often been strict rules about washing after menstruation — Bathsheba in the Old Testament was 'washing after her uncleanness' when David caught sight of her naked on her rooftop. The Old Testament book of Leviticus lists the rules about menstruation: 'And if a woman have an issue, and her issue in her flesh be blood, she shall be put apart seven days: and whosoever toucheth her shall be unclean until the even. . . . And whosoever toucheth her bed shall wash his clothes, and bathe himself in water, and be unclean until the even.' In societies where the mere sight of a menstruating woman was believed to be contaminating, women have sometimes been punished with death for failing to keep out of the men's way when menstruating.

These customs and beliefs may seem bizarre and cruel to us. Yet in our own society, girls are still brought up to be embarrassed about menstruation, to see it as dirty and to keep the evidence well hidden. Menstruation is still kept a secret from men in the family — from fathers and sometimes from husbands. Even in families where there is more openness, few men would willingly go into a shop to buy sanitary towels or tampons for their wives or girlfriends. Signs of menstruation, menstrual blood on your skirt, the tampon that will not flush away, are reasons for embarrassment. Recently, I bought a different brand of tampons. I took off the plastic wrapper, and found that there was no brand name on the box. Good, I thought, I can drop the box in my handbag and no-one will know ...

Since 1986, commercials for tampons and sanitary towels have been shown on Channel 4 television. These enigmatic commercials follow strict guidelines laid down by the IBA, which include a ban on any glimpse of the 'unwrapped article'. The coyness arises from fear of public protest. A six-month test of commercials for sanitary protection on ITV in 1980 resulted in over 1,000 letters of complaint. Every night on television, lots of sexual activity is described, discussed or depicted — but any direct mention of menstruation remains taboo.[7]

There are many theories about the origins of the taboo. Margaret Mead, the anthropologist, traced it to primitive people's fear of blood. Freud saw it as a response to men's fear of castration. Other writers have attributed it to male envy of women's creativity in giving birth, or to the meanings of bleeding for men, who only bleed when injured, never spontaneously. Whatever its origins, the taboo persists as a powerful force in our lives, shaping both our behaviour and our feelings about our bodies.

Some of these ideas about menstruation become embedded in attitudes to miscarriage. Like menstruation, miscarriage involves a lot of bleeding from the vagina; like menstruation, this bleeding is spontaneous. Consequently miscarriage is identified with the bleeding of menstruation, which is taboo, rather than with the bleeding that accompanies childbirth, which is not.

Miscarriage then brings together two of our most powerful taboos — death and menstruation. Is this why it remains such a hidden grief?

SOURCES

Colin Murray Parkes, *Bereavement*, Tavistock, London, 1972

REFERENCES

1. Pamela McDonald, 'Diary of a Miscarriage', *Irish Times*, September 1981
2. *The Baby Book*, Newbourne Publications Ltd, London, 1986
3. Pamela McDonald, *op cit*
4. Marina Warner, *Alone Of All Her Sex*, Picador, London, 1976
5. Ann Oakley, Ann McPherson and Helen Roberts, *Miscarriage*, Fontana, Glasgow, 1984
6. The Bristol Women's Studies Group, *Half The Sky*, Virago, London, 1979
7. *The Guardian*, 10 March 1986

7.
FINDING
COMFORT

Well, everyone can master a grief but [s]he that has it.
SHAKESPEARE, *Much Ado About Nothing*

In her novel *The Bell Jar*, Sylvia Plath uses the image of being
trapped in a glass jar to suggest what it is like to suffer
depression. Miscarriage, too, may trap a woman behind walls of
glass. She can see life going on as normal around her, but no-one
hears what she says, her questions go unanswered, her attempts
to say how she feels meet with denial and incomprehension. No
matter how hard she tries, she just cannot get through.

For the woman trapped behind walls of glass, it can be hard
to find comfort.

THE NEED FOR INFORMATION

After miscarriage, women are hungry for information. This
hunger can never be completely satisfied. An individual woman
is unlikely to discover what caused her miscarriage. However
there is still a lot she can learn, both about the possible causes of
miscarriage and about the emotional responses of other women.
Acquiring knowledge can be an important source of strength
after miscarriage. When asked where they found comfort, many
women put 'finding out all you can' at the top of the list.

Like a detective on the trail of a crime, a woman hunts for
clues, shifting through books and papers for anything that
touches on the subject that preoccupies her. Emily said, 'I read
every article, letter, book, I could lay my hands on. I scanned all
reading materials — even the daily newspaper — for the
smallest snippet of information about not only miscarriage, but
coping with grief, stillbirth and infertility.'

The word 'miscarriage' becomes a magnet that draws the
woman's eyes. She spends a lot of money on a glossy magazine

because this word appears on the cover, to find only a brief article on the subject inside. Or she acquires a whole heap of books on subjects like infertility and pregnancy loss. If she has friends in medicine, she urges them to tell her all they know.

Unfortunately this quest for information is not always successful. Because miscarriage is taboo, there is little information available, and hunting for information may take a kind of self-confidence which does not come easily to the woman who has suffered miscarriage. As Catharine put it, 'We spent quite a bit of time trying to find a book on the subject but had no luck. I never got up the courage to go and ask an assistant to order one of the ones I found out about. It's like admitting to a stranger that you've just had a miscarriage.'

EXPRESSING FEELINGS

We know that tears are good for us. The phrase 'a good cry' suggests that tears are valuable for people who are sad. The man or woman who comes to harm because he or she cannot cry at a grief is a familiar figure from fiction. As in Hans Anderson's tale 'The Snow Queen', being able to cry is a sign of psychological well-being — when Kay cries, his tears wash the glass splinter out of his eye and he is healed. But it is not always easy to cry. Those English virtues of restraint and self-control still shape our behaviour, and the woman who fears she is over-reacting after miscarriage will struggle to keep her tears inside.

Women's stories of how they cope after miscarriage re-affirm the value of expressing feelings in tears. Hazel said, 'This last time I've not been afraid of having a good cry. If I'm at work I just go to the loo. It helps a great deal, whereas before I thought I was being stupid and felt guilty and kept telling myself to "Pull myself together."'

Sadness is also expressed in words. In *Macbeth*, Shakespeare cautioned against the 'grief that will not speak' and advised 'Give sorrow words.' It is wise advice. By giving words to sadness, we can begin to free ourselves of it. Institutions as different as the counselling session and the Catholic confessional recognize the value of putting our sadness, anger and guilt into words.

Tessa contrasted her reactions after her first and second miscarriages. After the first one, she said, 'My closest friends visited regularly but it was some time before I could open up and talk about what had happened. People I knew on a casual basis, such as mothers at nursery, avoided me, and if they couldn't do that avoided the subject. I hated telling someone who didn't know that I'd miscarried. I'd watch their faces close up and then they wouldn't be able to look me in the eye, some would mumble platitudes and excuse themselves.' It was different after her second miscarriage. 'This time,' she said, 'I talked. Anyone expressing an interest got the full story. I opened up more and found to my surprise my closest friends were prepared to listen, some cried with me. As the weeks went by I talked out my grief and anger.'

Written words can help too. Some women have found it helpful to give their feelings a form by writing down the stories of their miscarriages, or making up poems about their lost babies. The story or poem has an existence in the world, separate from the woman who wrote it. Once it is written she can begin to distance herself a little from the experience she describes.

PARTNERS

Penny said, 'My husband is definitely the biggest support. He's not a complete angel, sometimes we've rowed about the situation, sometimes he loses his temper with me, but that's only natural and wouldn't be "him" if he didn't. The main thing is that he still loves me whatever I do, and when I'm really "down" cuddles me and makes me aware that he cares about me.'

For many couples, the weeks after miscarriage are a time of closeness. Women pay tribute to the good things their partners given them — support, comfort, patience, understanding. In these relationships, both partners seem able to talk about and understand each other's feelings.

But there is also another, sadder, strand in women's comments on men's responses. 'I had no-one who understood me, even my husband, who thought it was better never to mention it and act as if it had never happened.' 'My husband isn't sympathetic one bit, he just says snap out of it.' 'I think I'd feel better if Tom would talk about it, all he can say is it happened and there'll be others.' 'My husband just doesn't seem to understand, all I do is cry and am so depressed, that our marriage is nearly over.' For these women, the walls of glass that trap them after miscarriage separate them from their own husbands. The situation feeds on itself. The less the man seems to understand the woman's feelings, the more desperate she becomes for understanding. He implies she is over-reacting, this increases her loneliness, her loneliness adds to her unhappiness, and she alienates him further. It is a downward spiral that for some couples only ends with the end of the marriage.

OTHER PEOPLE

Pamela had a miscarriage at 21 weeks. She said, 'I went back to work about the time I would have gone on maternity leave. It was the single most difficult thing I've ever done in my life — facing everybody. In the six months I've been back at work nobody has mentioned the miscarriage once.'

Silence is one response. People may simply behave as though the miscarriage has not happened. Their silence tells the woman that what has happened to her is too terrible, or too embarrassing, shameful or unpleasant, to talk about.

Another frequent response is the stereotyped attempt to reassure. Other people may cope with their own pain and embarrassment about what has happened by trying to show that it was all for the best, or that it does not really matter so much — 'You're still young, you can have lots of babies', 'At 9 weeks it wasn't really a baby anyway', 'It's nature's way of getting rid of deformed babies', 'You're lucky, you can at least get pregnant', 'You can always adopt', 'You're better off without them', and so on.

Penny said, 'I was told all the usual things, but the one I hated most was "Well, it was probably grossly deformed." However true that may be I know my first baby would have been beautiful, warm, cuddly, smiling — all the things you hope a baby will be when he is eventually born.'

Many women are angry at the response they get from other people after miscarriage. Yet they also acknowledge that it is hard for other people to get it right. As Pamela pointed out, 'It's made me very demanding of people. I think I've judged them very harshly. I wanted them to acknowledge that something really awful had happened to me, but I don't know if I could have coped if they did.'

Unhelpful responses are so widespread that some women maintain it is not worth trying to talk about the experience to anyone who has not been through it themselves. But there is a kind of close friend who may prove an exception to the rule. Such a friend will accept your need to talk, and to go over your experience again and again. She will allow you to be sad and to cry. She will be able to cope with not having any answers herself and won't fall back on cliché comfort. And she won't expect you to be yourself again in a few weeks. Where women are lucky enough to have close loving friends, it does not seem to matter so much whether the friends know about the experience at first hand. Penny said of her friend, 'Although I don't think she quite appreciates all the heartache we've been through, she asks all the logical questions about it all and gives me plenty of opportunity to talk about it. She's never embarrassed by what I say.'

Perhaps surprisingly, family are often less than helpful. And there are many mothers who deal with their daughters' sadness by changing the subject if babies are mentioned, or ignoring every attempt their daughter makes to talk about the subject, something Tessa discovered. 'I found older relatives, especially my parents, did not want to listen. It seems that in days gone by miscarriage was a very taboo subject. My mother had suffered a miscarriage many years ago, but she told me to pull myself together and get on with life.' Hazel echoed this. 'Neither my mum nor elder sister [mother of three] ever experienced losing a baby and they couldn't understand why I was so upset. Both since then have admitted they wished they had never had children — my mum admitting to being jealous of me because she wishes she could have been a career woman.'

However this difficulty between mother and daughter is by no means inevitable. For Julia, her mother was one of the main sources of comfort after miscarriage. 'She was always there if I needed her either in person or on the telephone. She put up with tears and temper and would still love me and hug me after it all — whatever I'd said.'

SELF-HELP GROUPS

Most of the women whose stories appear in this book are either members of the Miscarriage Association or have at some time made contact with it. It is not surprising that for these women the Miscarriage Association comes high on the list of things that helped.

The Miscarriage Association is one of a number of self-help organizations that have grown up over the last few years, as people with health problems attempt to take back some control over their own health. The philosophy of self-help groups is to offer the people who join them both information and understanding. There is knowledge to be shared, as many women become experts on health problems that they have suffered themselves, and hopefully there will be empathic understanding of others with similar problems.

In the Miscarriage Association, support is given in various ways — through contact with individual women who offer support to others, through group meetings, and through a quarterly newsletter. Whichever form help comes in it is learning about other women's experiences that women find so valuable. Miscarriage is an isolating experience, and in this isolation a woman may wonder, 'Am I over-reacting? Do other women feel like this?' Reading or hearing other women's stories will answer these questions for her and give her permission to grieve. And some women find that involving themselves in other women's stories helps them come to terms with their own loss. Catharine said, 'One thing that did help was getting the Miscarriage Association newsletters and reading that what I was feeling was perfectly normal and experienced by hundreds of women before me. If it wasn't for the newsletters, I would be beginning to wonder if I was going round the twist. The baby would have been due last week and that has brought everything flooding back into the front of my thoughts, but I was prepared for that because of what I read in the newsletters.'

Self-help groups do not work for everyone. Pamela said, 'The woman who came to see me, asked me a lot of abrupt questions I didn't want to answer. It just wasn't right for me.'

Many women who join the Miscarriage Association at some point start offering support to others. Being the helper rather than the one who is helped is something you can only do once you yourself have to some extent recovered. However once a woman has reached that point, helping others may speed up the process of her own healing after miscarriage. Miscarriage feels like a terrible waste, but if you can use the insights you have gained to help others, some value can be salvaged from the experience. Putting your sadness to use can be therapy in itself.

COUNSELLING

Some women see professional counsellors or psychiatrists after miscarriage. For Lesley, the attempt to get professional help was a failure. Lesley suffered a missed miscarriage at 14 weeks. She recounts how: 'The experience, made worse by the attitude of the consultant, resulted in my becoming very depressed, to the extent that my GP referred me to a psychiatrist. I soon knew that the male psychiatrist didn't understand so I stopped seeing him.' Alison, on the other hand, found counselling helpful: 'Although I refused to take tranquillizers or sleeping tablets, I did go to see a counsellor at our Health Centre who encouraged me to let out some of my pain and grief and not to bottle it up.'

Counselling is not always of value — it can only be as good as the individual counsellor — but for women suffering intense distress after miscarriage, it can be helpful to 'give sorrow words' in a safe place with a sympathetic stranger.

If you would like counselling after your miscarriage, where can you turn? There is no pattern to counselling services. What is available depends on where you live. In some places you may be able to get free individual therapy through the NHS. For instance some health centres have a counsellor attached, and some clinical psychologists working in hospitals offer counselling to out-patients. If these services are available, your GP could refer you. There are also some counselling agencies that offer free sessions, and that you can approach direct. Your local Citizens Advice Bureau would advise you about this (their number will be in the telephone directory). If your miscarriage is causing problems in your marriage, you could consider contacting the Marriage Guidance Council.

If you do go to see your GP or a psychiatrist because you are depressed, you may be offered tranquillizers or sleeping pills. Tranquillizers are rather like aspirin — they alleviate the pain for a while, but they do not make you well. Many women nowadays are wisely very wary of such drugs. Sheila said, 'Never again would I so readily accept an offer of tranquillizers. They don't cure the cause of the grief, and they made me less capable of coping with day-to-day activities. Other interests within and outside the home would, I believe, have been more helpful in bringing life back to normal after a miscarriage, and might have prevented me becoming obsessed with my problems.'

For many couples, a counselling session at the time of the miscarriage might avert a lot of subsequent heartache. Judith had no counselling but would have like it. As she said, 'We both put brave faces on for each other and so totally missed how bad we felt. An independent outsider would have helped us I think.'

POSITIVE THINKING

Your attitude to your miscarriage is all important in your success in handling it and the subsequent grief. A time may come when you may feel a kind of acceptance of what has happened, like Carol. 'Four months after the ordeal I realize as soon as you can stop feeling sorry for yourself and asking why me? you can come to accept it.' Acceptance comes as you realize that nothing can change what has happened, and that it was not your fault or anybody else's. You would not want to forget your miscarriage — it has a place in your life — but you stop endlessly and obsessively going back over events to try and make them different, and you begin to let your lost baby go.

Letting go means thinking about the past in a different way. There are ways of thinking about the future, too, which may help women recover. Frances said, 'It helps to think positively and I am not going to give up hope of having my own baby.' What does it mean to 'think positively?' For Catharine, as for

Frances, it means holding on to hope. Catharine said, 'In the weeks as I recovered, one thing that I did do — which everyone except my husband thought was really daft — was to make some maternity clothes. As I hope to be pregnant again as soon as possible, I figured that I would need more clothes, so I might as well make them while I felt up to it. I feel I'm doing something positive towards the future, rather than dwelling on the past.' For Hazel, 'thinking positively' meant finding a way of thinking about her experience which filled her with gratitude rather than despair: 'When I feel depressed — which you can't help and comes over you quite quickly for no reason — I turn it into a feeling of joy that I was able to carry the babies and get to "know" them, and the joy they gave to Graham in the short time they were with us. It affects the way you look at your life in general and makes you appreciate your time together a lot more.'

For the woman who has suffered a number of miscarriages, holding on to the hope that she will finally achieve a successful pregnancy may start to seem unrealistic. Yet even in this situation there are ways of 'thinking positively'. Women can still think and act in ways that give them a sense of control over their lives. Judith has had five miscarriages, and said, 'We've pursued every treatment and felt we must make decisions for ourselves, not just let things happen: we'd requested tets, and we pushed for information, rather than let the hospital take over. I have also made a conscious decision to pursue adopting — a positive decision which has put me and us back in control of events in our lives.'

A PERSONAL PHILOSOPHY

Miscarriage, like any personal tragedy, can bring about a profound change in how you think about life. Most of us believe deep down that if we live our lives in the right way, then everything will turn out all right. Miscarriage challenges that belief. As it often happens quite early in a woman's life, it may prove to be a turning point, a first encounter with loss and death that sets her asking new questions.

You may find yourself thinking about death — your own and the deaths of people you love. You may question choices you have made in the past. You may wonder whether your work is as useful and significant as you thought. You may start to doubt whether you have any control over what happens to you. Once you start to think these disquieting thoughts, the world is no longer so safe and orderly a place.

In *Passages* Gail Sheehy describes just such a turning point.

For her it came when she witnessed the killing of a young boy in Belfast. 'Before then,' she says, 'I thought everything could be mended.'[1] After miscarriage, you know that there are things that cannot be mended.

Sheila went through thirteen miscarriages. She found her own way of coming to terms with this experience. 'Many people have thought me brave,' she recounts, 'to continue what seems a hopeless struggle. It wasn't bravery and I did give up after the twelfth miscarriage, but then I watched my grand-father die of cancer and, ill as he was, he fought hard for every precious day of life, and that convinced me that I could do the same for the life of my baby. Also, I have recently become a Christian and, whilst a religious faith of any kind is not everyone's "cup of tea", it has helped me to come to terms with life in general and possible childlessness in particular, and I no longer ask "Why me?"' For Sheila, religious commitment meant an end to some of the questioning. For another woman, there will be no answers, but the fact that she has asked those questions may change her priorities.

Some of the most urgent questions we ask ourselves after miscarriage concern the baby. Was my baby a person or just a cluster of cells? What is the meaning of a life which is ended before it is properly begun?

Theologians and philosophers down the centuries have speculated about the baby in the womb, about whether it is a person, and what rights it has, and at what point the soul enters the body. After miscarriage, we may find ourselves asking similar questions, but with an urgency that is missing from the theological debates. Clara lost her baby at 22 weeks. She asked, 'Where is he now? Thrown away physically, spiritually in heaven? If there is a God with a heaven and if Martin had a soul, then he's in the best possible place. If he didn't have a soul, then he was just a bunch of cells so it doesn't matter. So either way it's all right. After all, I wouldn't mind if my appendix was on the tip so if that's all he was, why should I mind? The fact that I mind like hell is entirely illogical. And anyway, I'm sure he's in heaven so it's just like someone dying, only worse, because I never got to know him. I just hope we'll recognize each other on Judgment Day.'

Occasionally, women have experiences which seem to touch on these questions. How we interpret such experiences, of course, depends on our own philosophy. Kim was carrying twins, but had a very early miscarriage at 7 weeks and one baby was born at term. After the birth she had to have a D & C. 'The surgeon said he removed the remains of my baby's twin ... I still wonder about her twin, but it is hard to mourn the loss of a baby near the beginning of pregnancy when one is still left with a baby at the end. Without thinking about it I sometimes feel that a baby is asleep somewhere in the house even when they are all awake, or that I have left someone behind when we all go out.'

Charlotte commented, 'Even though we have Matthew, who we both adore, we still feel "close" to our first son as though he is still with us. Neither of us is particularly religious, but we definitely feel he is still here, and it is a very comforting thought — to us at least.'

GIVING COMFORT — A NOTE FOR FRIENDS AND RELATIVES

Judy had a friend who lost her baby late in pregnancy and tells how difficult it was to offer any comfort: 'I saw her husband in the supermarket. I've read all those stories of people avoiding people who've lost a baby, and I've thought, how terrible. But you know when I saw him there I would have given just anything to be somewhere else. I had my back to him and I said to myself, "You've got to do it." So I went and said how sorry I was, but it was the most terrible effort.'

People who have been touched by tragedy stir up painful feelings in others. If your friend has suffered a miscarriage, you may feel helpless because you cannot make things right for her. You may want to distance yourself from her pain in case it invades you too. You may fear that you will lose control of your emotions and cry with her. Or you may feel a kind of hysterical laughter rising in your throat. Full of these unpleasant feelings, it is not surprising that we want to turn away. Shying away from other people's pain is as instinctive a reaction as flinching when we touch a hot surface. It is a response that counsellors in training spend a long time unlearning.

If your friend has had a miscarriage, the urge not to raise the subject at all when you see her may be enormous. All sorts of justifications may come into your head — 'Perhaps she's getting over it now', 'I don't know her that well', 'I don't want to remind her of it'. Yet if you don't talk about the miscarriage, your silence is still a message to your friend. You are telling her that what has happened to her is too terrible or embarrassing or disturbing even to be talked about. Many women who have miscarriages stress how painful they find the 'tactful' silence of people they know.

In his book on bereavement, Colin Murray Parkes says this about the first meeting between a person who has been bereaved and their friend: 'Pain is inevitable in such a case and cannot be avoided. It stems from the awareness of both parties that neither can give the other what he wants. The helper cannot bring back the person who is dead and the bereaved person cannot gratify the helper by seeming helped. No wonder that both feel dissatisfied with the encounter.'[2] It is like that with miscarriage too. You cannot put things right. There is nothing you can do that will give your friend her baby back, so you are bound to feel awkward, helpless, uneasy and embarrassed. There is no right way of handling the situation that will make these feelings go away. The best thing to do is simply to tell your friend how sad you are for her. Pamela said, 'There's this elderly man — he used to come to meetings at our house, I don't really know him very well at all — he came up to me in the street and took me by the arm and said, "I'm so sorry to hear about your miscarriage." I was very grateful for that.'

Sometimes women find attempts to reassure them after miscarriage unhelpful and even distressing. You want to make your friend feel better, and perhaps you come out with one of those standard reassuring remarks, 'You can always have another one', 'There must have been something wrong with it', 'It was only a little clump of cells.' These attempts to comfort make only the would-be comforter feel better. Try to avoid making remarks like this.

Sometimes people exercise great ingenuity in seeking out reasons why the miscarriage was not such a tragedy as the woman seems to think. Pamela remembers being told by a friend, 'Worse things are happening in El Salvador.' She was not comforted by this.

Your friend will probably want to tell her story over and over again. She may particularly need to go through the events that led up to the miscarriage. You may grow impatient because you feel these repetitions are pointless. You may feel that you should take control of the conversation and distract your friend from her sadness by getting her to think about more cheerful subjects, but what your friend is doing by going over her story is an important part of the process of mourning. By going through these things again and again, she is healing herself. You can help her by listening patiently when she wants to talk.

I have a picture of a stereotype social worker in my head — I hope a caricature. With head on one side and perpetually concerned expression, her response to any complaint from her client — the roof's leaking, the cat's been sick, the kids have mumps — is to ask, 'And how do you feel about it?' You don't of course want to be like that. You don't have to talk about the miscarriage and how your friend is feeling all the time. By all means try to cheer her up by suggesting a shopping expedition and a treat in a cafe. But if you are also able to be open to your friend's sadness, and if you don't shy away when she wants to talk, you will do a lot to help her to heal.

SOURCES

Colin Murray Parkes, *Bereavement*, Tavistock, London, 1972

REFERENCE

1. Gail Sheehy, *Passages*, Bantam Books, New York, 1977, p. 3
2. Parkes, *op cit*, p. 191

8.
MEN'S
FEELINGS

I staggered in the garage and handed them my heart.
Can you overhaul it cos the bloody thing won't start?
ADRIAN MITCHELL *Out Loud*

There are stories of men whose stomachs swell up during their
partners' pregnancies, or who have stomach cramps while their
partners are giving birth. This is called the 'couvade syndrome',
after the couvade ritual enacted by certain tribes, in which the
man mimes the act of giving birth while his wife is in labour.
The couvade syndrome is one pole of the experience of pregnant
fatherhood. At the other pole is complete detachment — the
man who impregnates the woman and leaves, or the still more
remote kind of fatherhood that has been made possible by
artificial insemination techniques. In between these two poles
are all the other kinds of expectant father, from the so-called
'new man' who learns the breathing exercises with his partner
and rubs her back during the birth, to the more conventional
man who is a 'good provider' but sees labour wards as strictly
female territory. For the woman carrying a baby inside her, her
role is given whether she likes it or not. But there are lots of
different ways to be a father.

It is no surprise, then, that in their experience of miscarriage
men vary a great deal. In women's stories of miscarriage there
are many common themes, but when I listen to men's stories, I
am much more aware of the contrasts.

DURING THE MISCARRIAGE

Peter recalls, 'Just as they were taking her out of bed they had
to stop and the baby was born then but I was not there, the
doctor had sent me down to his car to drive to hospital behind
the ambulance. They were a long time, but I waited in the car,

panicking and wondering what to do.' Waiting, panic, wondering
what to do — words that recur in men's descriptions of the
immediate experience of miscarriage.

Miscarriage can be frightening to witness. There may be a lot
of blood and the woman will be upset and in pain. Although it
rarely poses a risk to her health, miscarriage is a dramatic
event, which looks as though it might do the woman some
dreadful harm. In his helplessness, the man feels panic. He may
even fear that she will die.

In *A Kind of Loving*, Stan Barstow describes a man's
experience of miscarriage. The story has a vividly
autobiographical flavour. Vic has to marry Ingrid because he
gets her pregnant, then she miscarries. 'Is she going to die?. ...
Is this the way it's going to work out, with her dying and taking
the baby with her? And they say there's a pattern to life. A
plan. What plan?. ... I don't want her to die. I don't love her,
but I don't want her to die.'[1]

The man calls the doctor or goes to the hospital. Then comes
the waiting. Sitting by her bed, or separated from her — in the
car like Peter, by the telephone at home, or in a long bleak
corridor smelling of antiseptic. In an emergency a man may feel
a responsibility to take control and play an active part, but
when his partner miscarries, the man is left waiting helplessly
on the sidelines. He cannot take either of the active roles in this
drama. He cannot become the doctor and offer prognosis or pain
relief, nor can he take the woman's part and go through it for
her. He longs to do something to help, but there is nothing he
can do.

GRIEF

After miscarriage, some men grieve. Their grief has the same
themes as the grief of women. There is the sense of the
uniqueness of the lost baby. As John explained, 'I will never
forget our baby and when we do have one it won't replace the
one we've lost.' There is the jealousy of other couples for whom
it all seems to be so easy. Men, like women, ask, 'Why us?'
Geoffrey said, 'Why was it that people who were on the poverty
line could manage to go through pregnancy and perhaps be in
unhygienic surroundings and have no trouble and us, quite the
opposite, own house, good job, happiness, had to lose so many
babies ...?' And men who grieve also share with women that
pressing need to 'make it real'. David, for instance, wanted to
find out all he could about the baby: 'Afterwards, upon asking if
they could distinguish the sex of the baby, I was looked upon as
being silly and quickly dismissed and told, "It was just a little

clot." In *The Essential Father*, Tony Bradman describes the miscarriage which ended his wife's third pregnancy, and adds, 'Part of the reason I'm writing about it here is that I would like that lost child to have some sort of memorial; I still think quite often about him or her and what he or she would have been like.'[2]

But there is something else in men's accounts that is missing from the women's stories. These men assert their right to share in the sadness. Women worry about over-reacting, but men worry about reacting at all, and feel they have to justify their sadness and tears. Peter said, 'It was very painful for me and I can still feel weepy after all this time ... I do not think that men should not cry because that is part of grieving and as the baby had a joint start then both should be able to grieve.'

BEING STRONG

Sometimes, however, men do not show their feelings after miscarriage. As has already been mentioned, many women complain that their partners will not talk about the miscarriage, or show no feelings, or do not seem to understand.

In our society, feelings are female territory. Women are seen as more sensitive than men to the feelings of others, and as more likely to give way to certain feelings themselves — sadness and anxiety, for instance. In marriage, it is women who are responsible for the relationship side of life, both within and outside the family. Women bring up the children. Women maintain the family's emotional equilibrium — noticing who is sad or worried and finding out why. And often it is the woman who is seen as the 'emotional' partner, the one who 'worries', the one who gets 'worked up', the one who is, at times, 'neurotic'. When couples get into difficulties, it is the woman who complains that the man will not talk about their problems.

This is perhaps something of a caricature. Yet couples' responses to miscarriage often match the stereotype precisely. The woman longs to share her grief. The man shows no emotion, or won't talk about it, or doesn't seem to understand.

John was full of grief after his wife miscarried. 'When the doctor told me there was a chance she may lose it, I just felt as if my whole insides had collapsed. I still think about it every day, and I still feel that a part of my life has been taken away from me.' This is the language of grief that women use after miscarriage. John adds, 'I don't mention it much which upsets my wife. I have not been able to cry about it or show any other emotions.'

For John, it is not the feeling itself which is problematic, but his inability to express it. A man may wish he could let go, but simply is not able to. The habits of a lifetime are not easily given up. If you learned in the school playground that boys don't cry, you are not going to change suddenly now.

Robert said, 'When Anne came home I felt my job was to support her; she seemed completely battered both physically and emotionally. When she was upset I tried to reassure her and give her hope, when she was coping I thought it better not to grieve.' Robert suggests a second reason why men keep their sadness inside. Men may feel that, whatever their own feelings, they have to be strong for their partners. A man may feel that it is his role to offer a shoulder to cry on but not to cry and, by his strength and self-control, to keep things from falling apart. Sometimes it is only much later, once the woman's feelings have healed a little, that the man will say how he feels.

I wonder if men sometimes get this wrong. A woman who is distressed after miscarriage will long for some acknowledgement from her partner that he hurts too. If he doesn't react, she may think he isn't touched by what has happened. Sadness that is carefully contained can look like indifference. Self-control that is intended to hold things together, may form a wedge that pushes the couple apart.

MEN WHO DON'T GRIEVE

Alan tells a different kind of story:

> I didn't know anything about miscarriage before it actually happened to my wife. With the benefit of hindsight, I am almost inhibited about owning up to what my reactions were. In understanding what my wife was going through, I might just as well have been a Martian on a temporary visit to another planet. We do not yet have any children, and at 40, I have long since found all kinds of ways of filling my spare time. I was therefore in the position of the prospective father looking forward to the future not quite sure what was going to hit him, but from observation convinced it was going to be a total change. For this reason, my key reaction was simply relief. Once it was clear that things were not going as they should, apart from concern at my wife's distress, I just wanted to get the whole thing over with as fast as possible and forget about it — get back to normality. I cannot say I was sad.

Alan puts into words an ambivalence about pregnancy that

many men share. Plenty of men find their partners' pregnancies difficult, even hateful. Many of these men were keen on the idea before the pregnancy began, and will, when the time comes, make devoted fathers.

There may be small signs that something is wrong, little cracks in the smooth surface of life. One man refuses to talk about what to call the baby, another starts working late, another spends more time in the pub. Sometimes the situation is more serious — the man has an affair, or urges his wife to have an abortion, or simply walks out. Women who get beaten up by their husbands not infrequently report that the first assaults took place when they were pregnant.

When a man who has a close and caring relationship with his partner feels upset about the pregnancy, it will be a great source of guilt. Friends and relatives react to news of the pregnancy with delight and everyone expects you both to be thrilled. One man said it reminded him of childhood Christmasses which he had hated — the kisses from elderly aunts, the stodgy Christmas pudding, the interminable church services, the presents, less glossy and exciting than in the imagination, that had always broken by teatime, yet with everyone insisting, 'Aren't we all having a lovely time?'

What are the roots of these feelings about pregnancy? Alan hints at one of them. An older man who has settled into a way of life that suits him will have had plenty of opportunities to study the effects of child-rearing on his friends. After the birth of their first baby, they look worried and haggard, with shadows under their eyes. Their once immaculate home is littered with mucky discarded baby clothes, plastic objects in glaring colours and bowls of congealing cereal. They protest that they never have a moment to themselves, they are woken every night, they are always short of money, and they are too tired for sex. From where he stands, it is not an appealing prospect.

When he sees the effects of pregnancy on his partner, his apprehension seems to be justified. Particularly in the first few weeks of pregnancy, she is inaccessible, dreamy and wrapped up in herself. For Henry, the eldest of five, his partner's pregnancy reminded him of childhood. 'I hated my mother being pregnant. She went all giggly and sleepy. She wouldn't listen to me. She kept falling asleep when I wanted to tell her things I'd discovered, like why the sky is blue.' Seeing his partner preoccupied in this way, a man may feel that he is no longer so important to her. We all of us have a greedy infant inside that demands unconditional love. The man may fear that the child in him will no longer be cared for by his wife when there is a real child around.

His wife's pregnancy also confronts a man with the meanings of fatherhood. Fathers earn the family crust, they sit at the head of the table and carve the Sunday joint, they mete out punishment — 'Wait till your father comes home.' What does it mean to be the provider, the protector, the strong one? 'I don't want to be tied down,' says the stereotyped young man, shying away from marriage. It is an image of the responsibilities of fatherhood as chains or ropes that bind you and restrict your movements, restrictions that must be struggled against and resisted.

There may be worries about sex too. The opposition between sex and parenting is fundamental in our culture. Here for instance is sex expert Alex Comfort's arid version of the good life: 'The best modern sex is unproductive. ... The development of a recreational erotic life needs privacy. Sexual freedom just isn't compatible with a childbearing lifestyle.'[3] The opposition between sex and parenthood can be seen most clearly in our current images of motherhood. Mothers have a bad press in our society. Mothers have sensible shoes and scrubbed faces and talk about teething medicines and the price of mince. Mothers are neither intellectually or physically exciting. Sexual fulfilment then must be given up in exchange for the dubious delights of fatherhood.

Why is a man's understanding of pregnancy often dominated by fears about what must be given up? For the reality is that the woman gives up much more with the birth of a baby. A baby takes up far more space in a woman's life than in a man's.

There is, however, a crucial difference. Throughout pregnancy awareness of the baby growing inside her is forced on the woman. In the early weeks, sickness and tiredness tell her that dramatic changes are taking place inside her. Later, once the baby starts kicking, she has constant reminders of his or her presence and vigour. She knows she is harbouring a separate being inside her body, and she starts to relate to this new person before the birth. The man, on the other hand, may picture a new and less congenial lifestyle, without any sense of relationship with the central actor in it. He may think about what he will lose and not what he will gain. This is one reason why the loss of the baby in miscarriage may not touch the man as much. Vic in *A Kind of Loving* recognizes this: 'Somehow I can't care about the kid because it never really was a kid. It wasn't really anything except an egg growing in Ingrid; something that made us have to get married. It wasn't a person so I can't feel bad about losing it.'[4]

I wonder if there are also reasons that are more deeply hidden for the difficulties some men have with pregnancy.

Psychoanalysts have made much of the idea that women envy men for having penises, but there is little recognition of men's envy of women for the capacity to conceive, to grow fat with new life, and to give birth. Perhaps this envy also plays its part in men's responses to pregnancy and miscarriage.

This is what an Australian tribesman told an anthropologist about the origins of his tribe's fertility rites:[5]

> Really we have been stealing what belongs to them for it is mostly all women's business; and since it concerns them it belongs to them. Men have nothing to do really, except copulate, it all belongs to the women ... the baby, the blood, the yelling, the dancing, all that concerns the women; but every time we have to trick them.

The man who talked to the anthropologist saw clearly into the darker side of men's feelings about reproduction. In our own society 'womb envy' remains largely hidden, most apparent, perhaps, in certain attitudes within the medical profession — the enthusiasm with which some doctors seek to destroy women's reproductive capacities by performing unnecessary hysterectomies and the eagerness with which they appropriate those capacities through the new reproductive technologies. Perhaps 'womb envy' also explains why pregnancy can bring out the worst in the most devoted of husbands.

Some feminist writers have stressed how much the sexes have in common with one another. One inspiration behind this philosophy is the Androgyne, a figure from Greek myth, embodying both male and female characteristics in a beautiful completeness. The ideal of androgyny is an appealing one — and it has one kind of expression in sexual partnerships that are based on sharing, equality and understanding. But this ideal cannot quite encompass the experience of miscarriage. Our bodies are different, and because of that our experience of the world will be different too. Miscarriage confronts us with those differences. There are things which cannot exactly be shared. Some men are closely identified with their partners' experience, some feel out of touch, but none of them can know precisely what it means for a woman to lose a baby from inside her body. And so sometimes men and women are going to have very different responses to miscarriage. When that happens, there will be work to do.

Alan understood this only later. 'I suppose the key area where I would probably have reacted differently if I knew then what I know now is that I seriously underestimated the sheer sense of loss that my wife must have felt. I only saw it as a huge relief. I know now that she would have felt it more as a bereavement.'

GUILT AND SEX

After miscarriage, women feel guilty. Even women who do not feel the loss very keenly will ask themselves what is wrong with them or what they did to make this happen. Men are unlikely to share these doubts, but there are other kinds of guilt which men do feel.

There may be guilt because it is the woman who suffers the physical experience and the man cannot help her. Peter said, 'It must have been such an awful and painful experience. If I hurt as much as I did then she must be twice as bad.' There may be guilt about feeling the wrong things — the kind of guilt that Alan feels when he says, 'I am almost inhibited about owning up to what my reactions are.' And there may be guilt about sex. Men may feel guilty about making love because it led to conception and without conception there would have been no miscarriage. As Peter put it, 'I blamed myself for getting her pregnant again. I felt I had put her through an ordeal again when she should have been enjoying her first child. It put a strain on us both because I think Liz felt I should have been more responsible.' Men may feel guilty, too, because they made love during the pregnancy and they may blame themselves for causing the miscarriage. Sexual intercourse during pregnancy is thought by some doctors to involve a slight risk of miscarriage, but there is obviously a mismatch between the riskiness of sexual intercourse during pregnancy — which is minimal — and the guilt that becomes associated with it. The linking of sex and sin has a heavy weight of tradition behind it. We only too readily believe that sexuality is dangerous and that sexual pleasure will be followed by punishment. As it is often the man who takes the initiative in bed, perhaps he is the one who is most likely to feel this sense of guilt.

The woman may have her own reasons for being reluctant to make love in the weeks following the miscarriage. Grief and depression suppress desire. Miscarriage causes hormonal disturbances which may reduce libido. And miscarriage is a physical trauma, involving pain, internal examinations, perhaps a D & C under general anaesthetic, perhaps an induced labour. Many of her experiences of being touched during the miscarriage will have been painful or invasive. Now she says she 'doesn't want to be touched'. It may be a while before she can take pleasure in her body again. If she is desperate to conceive, yet unable to tolerate intercourse, it is a recipe for misery for both partners.

For most couples, these difficulties sort themselves out in time. A reluctance to make love for a while after miscarriage does not mean that anything is wrong with your relationship. After childbirth, it is very common for couples to wait a lot longer than the statutory six weeks before making love again. When you are grieving after miscarriage, a period of abstinence makes sense too. Knowing that this is quite common may help assuage those feelings of rejection that spring up so readily if one partner is more keen to make love than the other. In time, old feelings will re-assert themselves.

Occasionally a temporary reluctance to make love — on one or both sides — crystallizes into something more permanent. Myra said, 'Our sex life was never much good, to be honest. He was always more keen than me. After the miscarriage, he went off me, he just didn't want to know. We hardly ever made love after that. That summer our marriage broke up.' Where there are serious difficulties in a relationship, a miscarriage can be the stress that leads to breakdown.

COPING

No man I talked to mentioned other people as a significant source of help after miscarriage. Although none used the word, there must be a lot of loneliness for men after miscarriage.

It is often remarked that men do not have friends, or if they do they only talk about the football results and the latest in gear boxes. If this is true, it is one reason for the absence of helpful friends from men's stories. Another problem may be that very unpredictability of men's responses to miscarriage mentioned at the start of the chapter. Robert and Alan's experiences of miscarriage were very different, yet both found other people's reactions problematic.

Alan claimed that 'the most difficult reaction to cope with was other people's sympathy. It is nice to think there are so many kind people in the world, but I told as few as possible, because I didn't want a "sympathetic" response at the time, nor did I want to think about it particularly.'

Robert, on the other hand, said, '"How's Anne?" I am frequently asked, particularly by family and close friends when they enquire about Anne "since the miscarriage". No-one has ever asked me how I am coping, including my own family. I even talk sometimes about "Anne's miscarriages" which though physically accurate is not the way it feels. If a miscarriage is an emotional loss I've suffered too.'

SOURCES

Stan Barstow, *A Kind of Loving*, Black Swan, London, 1986
Tony Bradman, *The Essential Father*, Unwin, London, 1985

REFERENCES

1. Barstow, *op cit*, p. 252
2. Bradman, *op cit*, p. 108
3. Alex Comfort, *The Joy of Sex*, Simon & Schuster, 1972
4. Barstow, *op cit*, p. 254
5. Quoted in Paula Weideger, *Female Cycles*, The Women's Press, London, 1978

9.
DOCTORS

I do not like thee, Dr Fell.
The reason why I cannot tell.
But this I know and know full well,
I do not like thee, Dr Fell.
Nursery Rhyme

Miscarriage is a physical crisis which brings you into contact
with doctors and nurses and hospitals. The purpose of all the
medical care is to reduce the pain, the risks and the trauma of
miscarriage, and to support the woman through this medical
crisis. Yet women's accounts of their treatment at the hands of
the medical profession are the most disturbing parts of their
stories.

WOMEN'S COMPLAINTS

Some women complain about their treatment even in the weeks
before miscarriage. They feel that their worries were dismissed
and their doctors refused to listen to what they had to say about
the workings of their own bodies. Sylvia said, 'Within a few
weeks I began bleeding, but doctors continued to tell us that all
was well and I was just being neurotic. They took no notice of
the fact that I was losing large clots and when finally I begged
for a scan it revealed what I already knew — the baby was dead.
In fact the pregnancy had failed some 10 weeks before.'
    Once the miscarriage has started, women and their partners
complain that their feelings are overlooked or ignored. Rhona
commented that, 'When the doctor came to see me when I was
miscarrying the much wanted but unplanned baby, I was crying
and he said shortly, "It doesn't matter that much does it?"'
David, her husband, agreed. 'I was very upset at the way the
doctor spoke to my wife when I called him out in the middle of
the night. He did an internal straight away, told her that she
wasn't co-operating at all because of her crying and said she
might as well get rid of it.'
    During the miscarriage itself, pain relief may not be

adequate. Jean described waiting for pain relief from two
o'clock in the morning when she first asked for help, to three
o'clock in the afternoon: 'All this time I had no pain relief in
case the fetus was viable and no food in case it wasn't and I had
to have a D & C.' Teresa Kewley, in an article published in
Spare Rib, tells a similar story: 'Later that night, after hours of
contractions, I asked for pain-relief from the nurses because I
was finding it impossible to bear the pain. They offered me two
panadol! (And no water to swallow them with since I was
shortly due to go to theatre.) Eventually I cried so much that
they gave me an injection, but only after I begged for it.'[1]

Women who suffer missed miscarriages seem to be
particularly unhappy with the way the situation is handled.
Many women describe their distress at being sent home with a
dead baby inside them, to see if they expel it themselves, or to
wait until a bed is available for a D & C. Susanna said, 'Being
sent home with my dead baby inside me was terrible. By the
next day, Saturday, I could stand it no longer, and started the
labour off myself by lifting a heavy laundry basket — foolish I
agree. In the late afternoon I started losing blood.' (It is of
course very unlikely that the bleeding started because of what
Susanna did. Contrary to popular belief, there is no evidence
that heavy lifting causes miscarriage.)

Perhaps the most common complaint of all is about the use of
the term 'abortion'. In everyday language 'abortion' means the
ending of a pregnancy at the mother's request, but in medical
terminology it describes a very different experience, the
spontaneous loss of a much wanted baby. Women have strong
feelings about this usage. Many say they hate it. They hate it
because of the meaning it has for them as non-medical people.
As Vera expressed it, 'I was told I had had an incomplete
abortion, which made me feel I was to blame.' Women also hate
the term for the effect it has on others. Rose said, 'When the
night staff passed notes to the day staff while standing at the
bottom of my bed, she stated, "This is the lady for the
abortion." All around me other ladies looked disgusted at me for
wanting an abortion — but my baby was most wanted.' Marian
recounted a similar experience: 'One nurse thought I was having
an abortion and started to give me a lecture which made me
hysterical again, as she was telling me how selfish I was as some
people who wanted a baby couldn't have one.' Over 80 per cent
of women who responded to a Miscarriage Association survey on
medical treatment felt the term 'miscarriage' should always be
used.

Other terms some medical staff may use can also cause
distress. Emily said, 'The following explanation of a D & C

given to me upset me a great deal — "Please sign this form; it's to enable me to evacuate your uterus. This means I will just do a quick and simple scrape away of the lining of your uterus. It's necessary, you see, to clean you up so that you can start again." Perhaps I'm too sensitive but I was upset to hear the doctor was going to scrape away my baby. I wanted it to be saved, not discarded. I was angry that he should suggest my insides were "dirty" — I certainly didn't feel I needed to be "cleaned up". Strangely not one doctor or nurse ever suggested that a baby was involved in the whole process of miscarriage and D & C.'

The insensitive organization of wards in some hospitals is another cause for complaint, as Sheila discovered. 'Every time I was hospitalized for miscarriage, there were one or more women in the same ward (sometimes in neighbouring beds) undergoing induced abortion. Their cheerfulness and my anger at the termination of healthy pregnancies and what I considered the immoral taking of life, confused my emotions still further.' Sheila speaks for a lot of women. For the woman who is going through a miscarriage, being put in the same ward with women who have chosen to have abortions can be a source of intense distress.

Over and over again, it seems, there is no recognition of the meaning of the experience for the woman or her partner. This insensitivity is apparent in the way news is broken of what has happened. Janice recalls, 'When my husband came to the hospital after getting the message wrong and thinking I was all right, the sister on the desk said, "What are you doing here?" He said he thought I was coming home. She just looked at him and said in front of all the other nurses, "The baby is dead."' Elizabeth's experience was equally harrowing:

At 14 weeks I had a scan. The consultant sat at one end of the room whilst I was scanned. Obviously something was wrong as three observers twiddled all sorts of knobs. When I asked if the baby had died the 'scanner lady' told me it wasn't her job to tell me, whereupon the consultant lifted his head and said, 'Tell her to come back in a fortnight.' I returned after two weeks with my husband and was rescanned in silence. I got dressed and was sent to another room to see the same consultant who told me, 'Yes, well, the scan confirms what we saw two weeks ago. Come back next week for a D & C.' When we asked what that meant he said, 'Well, your pregnancy has ended.' As far as he was concerned that was that. As I then started crying, he said it wasn't worth his effort talking to me as pregnant women are all over-emotional and rather neurotic and I was then ignored.

Many women complain about the lack of adequate aftercare in the weeks following miscarriage. Some hospitals offer follow-up appointments six weeks after the miscarriage, but others do not. This was Debbie's experience at a hospital that did:

> I had never seen the consultant before and was still trying hard to understand what had actually happened to me and my baby. He told me, 'You probably flushed it down the toilet' — I hadn't — and seemed unable to explain, as my GP later did, that the fetus had probably disintegrated. I was searching for reasons as to why it had happened to me and asked lots of questions but the answers were vague and ill-informed, along the lines that 'nothing was known' and 'it was very common.' When I asked about the possibility of cervical incompetence, I was told, 'I'm sure you have a perfectly beautiful cervix.' I was unclear on what evidence this was based.

When aftercare is offered, the setting as well as the content of the consultation may be far from ideal, as Melissa pointed out. 'They hold the gynae clinic in the ante-natal clinic, with all those pictures of babies and breastfeeding on the walls. I cried my eyes out.'

A lot of hospitals, however, do not offer any follow-up appointments after miscarriage. Women may hope for some aftercare from their GPs and receive none. Dorothy said, 'I feel so disappointed that my own GP, who until now has always showed such concern for myself and my family, should not even send a health visitor on a routine visit to see whether I'm coping or not. I find myself thinking, if others don't attach very much importance to miscarriage, then why on earth can't I forget the whole thing?'

Some women arrange to visit the GP themselves. They frequently complain of a lack of information and failure to answer their questions. 'You have to wrench information out of them,' said Pamela. 'I do wish doctors would say "I don't know" when they don't know,' commented Rachel. Sometimes women feel they know more about miscarriage than their GPs. Ruth said, 'I registered with a new GP and asked to be referred to St Mary's. The GP refused saying, "You can't go running all over the country after a fairy story in a woman's magazine."'

In the GP's surgery, as in the hospital, the meaning of the experience to the woman may be ignored. Patricia wrote, 'Although I have confidence in the doctor who is treating me, he doesn't appear to have the time to give me much information and the only time I tried to express my feelings to him, I was offered a prescription for Valium which I neither need nor want.' Emily had a similar experience: 'My GP's apparent lack of concern hurt me deeply. I know that miscarriage is common but this was the loss of my baby not any baby. I wish that he could have said, 'I'm sorry ... you must be feeling very sad about this.'''

Women's complaints make grim reading. It is clear that many women who suffer miscarriages are being very badly served by their health service.

This matters a great deal. It matters in the immediate aftermath of miscarriage. Miscarriage often stirs up deep feelings. Sometimes sadness crystallizes into depression, but sensitive care at the time of the miscarriage may help a woman to cope in the following months. Some women with experience of several miscarriages point to one good hospital experience, and explain that on that occasion they did not get depressed because the care they received in hospital made all the difference.

Treatment at the time of the miscarriage also has implications for the future. According to the Swedish study already mentioned, women with a history of recurrent miscarriage who were given 'optimal psychological support' during pregnancy had a much improved chance of carrying their pregnancies to term.[2] The foundations for this kind of care could well be laid in the follow-up to the previous miscarriage. Yet, far from laying these foundations, some doctors are actively undermining the confidence of their patients who suffer miscarriages.

So what can be done to improve medical responses to miscarriage? One of the striking things about women's stories is that they are complaining about simple and obvious failures and mistakes. They complain that no-one answered their questions, that no-one said, 'You must be feeling upset.' Women are not asking for elaborate and expensive reforms.

Listed below are a few of the very simple changes that women would like to see.

LEARNING TO UNDERSTAND

The woman who is miscarrying needs understanding from the medical staff who care for her. She needs them to allow her to be sad and to recognize and respect her need to grieve.

In order to do these things, medical staff have to be able to cope with their own feelings about miscarriage. The loss of a baby in its mother's womb is disturbing for those who care for the woman. There is the pain of her loss, and of not being able to do anything to prevent it. There may also be other feelings, even harder to express — feelings of horror or disgust. An editorial on stillbirth in *The Lancet* comments 'Death in utero is extraordinarily chilling and repugnant . . .', and refers to a study which showed that 'in cases of stillbirth doctors are compulsively reluctant to know, notice or remember anything about these patients. . . . The whole subject of stillbirth is somehow abhorrent to the medical profession.'[3]

Doctors have little or no training in dealing with these feelings. So they learn to cope with their encounters with pain and death, and with the sexual meanings of gynaecological procedures, by cultivating a detached manner. The word 'clinical', which originally meant 'of the sick-bed', is now used to describe this detached manner. The word is often paired with 'cold'.

Yet in spite of the obstacles presented by their training, some doctors manage to convey tremendous warmth. Rowena said, 'My consultant was marvellous — almost as upset as I was. He telephoned my husband when we found the baby had died and took me to his secretary for a cup of coffee and gave me a big hug as I left and said he just didn't know what to say as he had been so sure it would be all right.' Some doctors, like Catharine's understand because of what they have been through themselves:

> The doctor was a tremendous help to me, the first time I went to see him, about a week after it happened, I was absolutely desolate, I couldn't tell him about it I was so upset, but as it transpired he had lost his own newborn baby in a cot death only three weeks previously. He just shrugged his shoulders with his eyes full of tears and said, 'It's not bloody fair, is it.' I wanted to hug him, our loss seemed trivial in comparison. I felt dreadfully guilty, yet much better for talking to him.

Not everyone is like Rowena's consultant, who seems to have been a naturally warm and caring person. And not everyone learns the hard way, like Catharine's doctor. But even those who have reserved temperaments, and who cannot draw on their own experience, can learn to be empathic. Sensitivity to other people's feelings is not a mysterious gift. It can be taught.

Sheila gives a vivid picture of a ward where all the medical staff had learnt to be sensitive to the emotional needs of women who miscarry. After her thirteenth miscarriage, she went to a new hospital:

This experience was totally different to all the others. I was encouraged to talk and to cry, not only by my partner but by each of the doctors and nurses who attended me with the utmost kindness. My questions were invited and, where possible, answered, and cups of tea, cuddles and hankies were readily available even at four in the morning! In those few days I was able to grieve not just for that baby but for them all. At last I was able to talk openly about losing a child which was 'disposed of' without prayers or flowers, and the bleakness of my past and my future. Years of anger, hurt and tears flowed over countless shoulders day and night, so that when I left the hospital I was able to put it all in perspective.

THE FETUS IS A BABY

Recognition of what the fetus means to the woman is one aspect of 'understanding.' This recognition has practical implications.

Seeing her baby can help a woman to recover after miscarriage, as it gives her a focus for her sense of loss. Medical staff should always offer the woman a chance to see what has been miscarried. If she can see her baby, this may be a comfort to her. If there is nothing clear to see, at least this will do away with the fantasy that she has been carrying something ugly or deformed inside her body. Not every woman will want to look, but the opportunity should be offered.

Hospital staff should also record as much as possible about the baby. Women often want to know the sex of the baby. Where possible the woman should be told and the sex recorded in her medical notes.

In recent years, there have been changes in the hospital management of stillbirth. In many hospitals, photographs are taken, so that even when the woman or her partner did not want to look at the time, they can change their minds later. This practice should be extended to miscarriages after 14 weeks.

With recognition of the meaning of the experience for the woman, the management of missed miscarriage would change. Women are often sent home knowing they have a dead baby inside them. The doctor may be waiting to see if the woman will miscarry without being induced, or simply waiting until a bed becomes available. This situation causes great distress to the woman. A missed miscarriage requires an immediate medical response, whether it be D & C or induction of labour.

CHANGES IN MEDICAL LANGUAGE

The term 'spontaneous abortion' should be dropped in favour of 'miscarriage'. This is the simplest but also the most universal recommendation made by women who have miscarried.

Greater insight on the part of doctors into the meaning of miscarriage for women would hopefully lead to other changes in language too. There would be fewer references to, for instance, 'having that lot scraped out' or the need to 'clean you up so you can start again'. Doctors might start to listen to the words that women themselves use to describe their experiences, and attempt to share in their language — to talk about babies who have died, rather than 'products of conception' that need to be 'evacuated'.

EFFECTIVE PAIN RELIEF

Miscarriage can be very painful — it may hurt as much as full-term labour — but if you are miscarrying you cannot draw strength from knowing that the pain is leading up to the moment when you can hold your baby. Women who are miscarrying should be offered the best possible pain relief.

Doctors are not very good at treating patients who cannot be cured. Western medicine puts the priority on intervention. Surgery is the most glamorous branch of medicine whereas the provision of good symptomatic treatment for patients whose predicament cannot be changed is much less valued. But the fact that the doctor's skill cannot prevent the miscarriage is no reason for him or her to walk away. The woman who is miscarrying cannot be cured, but she does need to be cared for — and that means skilful pain relief.

ORGANIZATIONAL CHANGES — WARDS AND CLINICS

Women who have miscarried may find themselves in wards with women who have chosen abortions, or where they can hear newborn babies crying, and they may have follow-up appointments in clinics full of pregnant women. Many women have asked for greater sensitivity in the organization of wards and clinics.

These recommendations bring us up against the issue of resources. The NHS is grossly over-stretched and, in the absence of adequate resources, it may not always be possible to organize wards and clinics to cater to women's emotional needs. However it is still important that medical staff and administrators should recognize that there is a problem. With imagination, they may be able to come up with solutions, even in the present difficult circumstances of the NHS.

SUPPLYING INFORMATION

Women and their partners should be given as much information as possible at the time of miscarriage. They need answers to questions like these: What causes miscarriage? What physical after-effects can I expect? Will it happen again? Is there any treatment? What can I do to give myself the best possible chance next time? They also need information about the possible emotional effects of miscarriage, and they need to know where to get help — the addresses of local support groups and the Miscarriage Association, for instance.

Doctors justify medical secrecy by saying that patients may need to be protected from frightening information. With some kinds of information, a case can be made for discretion, for instance, a doctor may decide — rightly or wrongly — to protect a patient from the knowledge she or that he has cancer. In the case of the woman who has miscarried, this justification collapses like a house of cards. There is nothing to protect the woman from. The miscarriage has already taken place.

FOLLOW-UP APPOINTMENTS

Hospitals should routinely offer follow-up appointments six weeks after the miscarriage. A follow-up appointment is a chance for the woman and her partner to ask more questions, to talk about their feelings since the miscarriage, and to be given advice on pre-conception care. At present, follow-up is by no means routine and when it is offered it rarely fulfils these functions.

There is one question that worries almost every woman who miscarries: Is there something wrong with me which makes another miscarriage likely or inevitable? Tests can sometimes give answers to this question. Tests are usually postponed until the woman has miscarried three times, but many women argue that tests should be carried out after one miscarriage.

The reasons for postponing tests do make sense. Both tests and treatments are quite limited in their scope. Tests may sometimes, but by no means always, show what is wrong. But even if a woman was given a whole battery of tests after one miscarriage, and a possible reason for her miscarriage was found, she would still probably not be offered any treatment. None of the treatments available for miscarriage is without risk. Also women with various problems which make them more likely to miscarry, such as abnormally shaped wombs, do often carry pregnancies to term without any treatment. So it rarely makes sense for a doctor to rush in and treat after one miscarriage. In other words, you may be missing out on information as a result of not being tested, but you almost certainly will not be missing out on treatment.

Clearly there is a need for doctors to be flexible. If, for instance, cervical incompetence is suspected, treatment after one miscarriage is essential. If a woman is not offered any tests after miscarriage, she should still be told what tests are available, and why they are not being done as yet.

AN END TO BEING PATRONIZED

Women who are miscarrying or have miscarried should be treated as intelligent adults with valid emotions.

There is a picture of a pregnant woman which is used to advertise a drug in the medical journals. She is blonde, baby-faced, dressed in white broderie anglaise and has the innocent trusting eyes of a child. It is a curious misrepresentation of pregnancy, a time when few of us feel innocent or immaculate. Perhaps a figure from a Beryl Cooke painting might be more appropriate. This picture sticks in my mind. I wonder if this fair-haired child-woman is, for many doctors, the perfect pregnant patient. A patient who is trusting and totally un-curious. A patient who never asks questions, never informs herself, never makes demands and, if things go wrong, certainly never embarrasses the doctor by getting upset.

To the qualities of the perfect patient I should perhaps add illiteracy. I once queried some treatment I had been given, in response the consultant patted my pregnant stomach and said benignly, 'Never read books, dear, whatever you do, never read books.' In his book on pregnancy, Gordon Bourne insists that your doctor — and presumably Gordon Bourne's own book — should be your only sources of information. He has a whole page headed 'Don't read medical text books' and warns, 'Do not settle down to some good solid reading about a rather frightening complication that you imagine might be affecting you.'[4]

Many of the women whose stories I have quoted were treated dismissively by their doctors. If they failed to conform to the image of the perfect patient by starting to cry because they had lost their babies, they were called 'neurotic', 'over-emotional', or accused of 'not co-operating', or they were offered addictive tranquillizers. If, confused by the lack of information they were given, they tried to inform themselves by asking questions, they were patronized, as when Debbie asked about the possibility of cervical incompetence and her consultant replied, 'I'm sure you have a perfectly beautiful cervix.' That kind of remark must be familiar to most women who have seen doctors about pregnancy or miscarriage. Such remarks can fill you with helpless anger, because it is very hard to oppose a man whose refusal to take you seriously is disguised as chivalry.

MORE RESEARCH

Research into miscarriage should be made a higher medical priority.

In a lot of recent discussion about women and medicine, medical 'technology' has been opposed to what is 'natural'. Much of this discussion has been about labour and childbirth, as women assert their right to choose the kinds of birth they want. And in this context 'technology' has come to be seen as bad, and the 'natural' as good. There has been a fashionable fantasy about the good old days when men with their nasty instruments had nothing to do with obstetrics — a fantasy about wise women with their herbal infusions and secret knowledge, about women in tune with their bodies, aided in childbirth only by the midwife's skilful hands.

These simple oppositions are unhelpful. Medical technology — in spite of its lapses — has brought great benefits. And many women who have miscarried are all for medical technology. In fact we want more of it — more research, more interventions, more treatment options.

Why is there so little interest in miscarriage on the part of doctors? Why, with just one or two exciting exceptions, do medical researchers simply ignore its existence? The reasons for this silence surrounding miscarriage have already been discussed. Doctors, of course, share in the values and attitudes of the wider society and these walls of silence hem in their thinking too. But the lack of interest in miscarriage on the part of the medical profession can also be seen as part of something wider — the low priority given to those health problems that only affect women. There are a number of problems that present no risk to life, yet cause pain and distress to millions of women: pre-menstrual tension, period pain and menopausal problems among them. Conventional medicine offers virtually nothing for any of these problems and seems to show little interest in researching them. The lack of concern presumably has its roots in one fact: these things never happen to men.

MORE WOMEN DOCTORS

To all the recommendations voiced by women or implicit in their stories, I want to add another more general one. We need more women to make their careers in obstetrics and gynaecology.

Gynaecology — 'the science of women' — is the branch of medicine in which women should logically predominate. Yet there is a much lower proportion of women in gynaecology than in certain other branches of medicine.

The fact that a doctor is a woman, of course, does not make her necessarily woman-centred. She will absorb inevitably some of the values of her training and of her colleagues — and medicine is a thoroughly male business.

A doctor, once qualified, starts his career by working preposterous amounts of overtime for a year. It is a kind of macho initiation ritual reminiscent of the ritual wounds or period of starvation a male adolescent may have to endure in some tribal societies in order to achieve manhood. Once initiated, the young doctor who stays in hospital medicine finds himself caught up in an aggressively competitive career structure. Relationships with colleagues are based on competitiveness rather than mutual support, and consultants expect subservience from those below them. In this atmosphere, in which it becomes almost impossible for doctors to support one another, the favoured emotional style is the typically male one of restraint and objectivity. 'Feminine' feelings, like distress or anxiety, have to be suppressed. The priorities of medicine as a whole could be seen as 'masculine' too. The emphasis is on active intervention, heroic surgery and the use of exciting new technology. The doctor's job is to cure, while the caring role in hospitals is relegated to nurses — who are poorly paid, low in status and mostly female. Caring is defined as a female and secondary concern.

It is hard for a woman doctor to challenge all this maleness. However, do not think it is romantic to believe that an increase in the numbers of women working in obstetrics and gynaecology might shift some of the priorities. Women doctors are more likely than men to have been touched by all the questioning there has been in the last twenty years about the place of women in society, and particularly about women's health needs. Women doctors are less likely than men to have patronizing and dismissive attitudes to women. A survey of medical students' attitudes found that male students were significantly more likely than female students to stereotype women in a negative way.[5] Because of their experience of their own bodies, women doctors are compelled to question the more bizarre theories held by some male doctors. If you have had period pain yourself, you are less likely to attribute it to some profound psychological inadequacy. In particular, some women doctors will have personal knowledge of miscarriage. As one woman doctor confessed, 'I've behaved very differently towards my miscarriage patients since I had one myself.'

CHANGING YOUR DOCTOR

A blueprint for change is of no immediate help to you if you are unhappy with the medical care you are receiving now. In the short term, your only option is to change your doctor. The procedures are quite simple, but it does take a certain amount of self-confidence to make this decision. Remind yourself that the health service is there to serve you, and that you and your baby have a right to good medical care.

If you want to change your GP you do not have to see your GP to tell him or her. Instead you can send your medical card to your local Family Practitioner Committee (England and Wales), Local Health Board (Scotland) or Central Services Agency (Northern Ireland). You should state in a covering letter that you want to change your GP, but you do not have to give a reason. They will return your card with a slip which allows you to transfer not sooner than two weeks and not more than six weeks after they received it. You should then complete part 1 of the slip and take it to your new doctor who will sign your card and send it to the Family Practitioner Committee for replacement. If you have lost your card, you should write to the FPC and explain the situation.

If you want to change your consultant, you could discuss this with your GP and see whom he or she recommends. Or you could find the name of a consultant whom other women have found helpful. Other women who have had miscarriages will be the best source of information on the subject and your local Miscarriage Association contact would probably know about women's experiences locally. Take the name to your GP and ask him or her to refer you.

The changes that many women want to see in medicine — changes in the response to all women's problems which would include changes in the treatment of miscarriage — sometimes seem very slow in coming. Yet in recent years, some progress has been made. In many hospitals, women are given more control over labour, and stillbirth is managed in a more sensitive way. Things may be changing, too, in the response to miscarriage. The distressing experiences of medical care described in this chapter are not universal. It is well worth seeking out better care, for there are doctors around who are starting miscarriage clinics, instigating research, listening to women. Perhaps a little guarded optimism is finally in order.

REFERENCES

1. Teresa Kewley, 'Miscarriage', *Spare Rib*, April 1985
2. B. Stray-Pedersen and S. Stray-Pedersen, 'Etiologic factors and subsequent reproductive performance in 195 couples with a prior history of habitual abortion', *American Journal of Obstetrics and Gynaecology*, vol. 148, no. 2, 15 January 1984
3. Editorial, *The Lancet*, 4 June 1977, p. 1188
4. Gordon Bourne, *Pregnancy*, Pan, London, 1975, p. 2
5. Wendy Savage and Pat Tate, 'Medical students' attitudes towards women: a sex-linked variable?' *Medical Education*, 17, 1983, pp. 159-64

10.
LOOKING FORWARD

And the angel of the lord appeared to the woman and said
to her, 'Behold you are barren and have no children; but
you shall conceive and bear a son. Therefore beware, and
drink no wine or strong drink, and eat nothing unclean, for
lo, you shall conceive and bear a son.'
(Judges 13: 2-3)

Perhaps you have a picture in your mind's eye. There you sit in
a hospital bed, smiling, surrounded by cards and flowers, your
tiny baby in your arms. In the months after miscarriage, the
chances of turning this enticing picture into reality seem remote.
First, there is the obstacle course of your next pregnancy to
negotiate.

HOW LONG TO WAIT?

'When can I try again?' is one question that almost every
woman who miscarries asks her doctor. There may be
uniformity about the question. There certainly isn't any about
the answers, as these women found out: 'Everyone had different
advice — everything from "Wait till you get home" to "a year at
least".' 'I had totally confusing advice from three sources —
three months, six months, after two periods.' 'Some doctors said
wait three months, others said try immediately. All the nurses
on the ward said to try immediately.' It is quite a mixed bag of
answers. None of them is 'right'; nobody knows the best gap to
leave, because no research on the subject has been done. As so
often when there are no certainties, opinion gets dressed up as
fact. Doctors, used to telling people what to do, turn guesses into
instructions. Women are rarely told where these instructions
come from or whether they have any scientific basis. It is very
confusing if you are on the receiving end.

However there is some research on pregnancy outcomes following full-term pregnancy which throws a little light on this topic. The research shows that getting pregnant again very soon after having a baby increases the risk that the next baby will be of low birth-weight, and low birth-weight babies are more likely to die around the time of birth.[1] On the basis of this research, the World Health Organization has recommended that women leave an interval of at least 18 months between the beginnings of pregnancies.[2] In other words, it is best to wait at least nine months after the birth of a full-term baby before trying to conceive again.

It is not clear why this should be so, but the most likely explanation is that the woman's body takes a while to adjust after childbirth. Pregnancy involves a huge upheaval in a woman's system — in her biochemistry, her immunology, her circulation, her hormones. During pregnancy, too, the woman's system may be depleted of essential nutrients that go to sustain the baby. Leaving a gap allows time for those stores to be replenished.

The same factors will be operating to some extent after miscarriage too. Even when pregnancy is interrupted by an early miscarriage there will have been profound changes in a woman's hormone levels and essential nutrients may have been used up by the hard work of sustaining the fetus. So after miscarriage, too, you may give the next pregnancy a better chance if you leave a gap before trying to get pregnant again.

However there are different kinds of miscarriage. A pregnancy that lasts five months will stress your body more than one that is lost at seven weeks. Some doctors advise leaving three months after an early miscarriage, and rather longer after a late miscarriage, perhaps a month for every month the pregnancy lasted — a five month gap after a miscarriage at five months, for instance.[3] In view of what we know about birth spacing after full-term pregnancy, this advice makes sense.

But miscarriage isn't only a physical event and there may well be other reasons for leaving a gap before the next pregnancy. Women often talk about the urge to replace the lost baby, almost as though the past could be cancelled out and re-enacted in a different way. We may feel that only by having another baby can we put the world to rights again, and recover what we have lost. Yet at the same time we know that the world is not like that — the lost baby cannot truly be replaced. When we choose a name for an unborn baby, however early in pregnancy, and then the baby is lost, we will be unlikely simply to pass on the same name to the next baby. We recognize the uniqueness of the baby in the womb, however tiny he or she may be.

Leaving a gap gives you time to grieve. Once you have grieved for a while, you can let your lost baby go, and get ready to welcome a new one in all his or her uniqueness. And once you have started to recover, you will be strong enough to cope with any difficulties you may have to face in the next pregnancy.

So there seem to be a number of good reasons for waiting three months if you had an early miscarriage, and longer if the miscarriage was in the second trimester. But good advice is not always easy to follow. The waiting may be hard to do. Caroline said, 'I found using contraceptives most unpleasant. I wanted to make a baby, not prevent one.'

There is one way to make the waiting a little easier. If you put the time to good use and spend it preparing for your next pregnancy, the waiting may be easier to bear. By thinking about your lifestyle and improving your diet, you can make this waiting time work for you. You will have started caring for your next baby even before you conceive.

THE CASE FOR PRE-CONCEPTION CARE

Fran spent four months preparing to run a marathon. She put herself on a carefully worked out training programme, including running every day with warm-up exercises first. On Sundays, she did a longer run, a little further each week. Two weeks before the marathon, she started to wind down, doing shorter runs. For a week before, she stuffed herself with pasta, so she would have plenty of calories to burn when she 'hit the wall'.

With sport, we take this kind of preparation for granted — the regular workouts, the planned build-up to the marathon or big match, the careful choice of equipment (Fran travelled 60 miles to find the right pair of running shoes). The preparation includes attention to diet — minimal diets for jockeys, huge platefuls of red meat for the boat crews in Oxford and Cambridge colleges, 'carbohydrate loading' for marathon runners like Fran. It may also include early nights and abstinence. High-status sportsmen suspected of indulging in drugs and sex while on tour may be accused in banner headlines of letting their country down.

But what about pregnancy — which takes a far greater toll on our bodies, and where the stakes are far higher than in any sporting event? If you go to the doctor and say you are planning to get pregnant, he will probably send you away and tell you to come back when you are pregnant, so he can fix up an ante-natal appointment for you. He may add that it is a good idea to give up smoking. If you tell him you have had one or even two miscarriages, you will probably get the same response.

This nonchalant approach to the start of pregnancy has been strongly opposed by some doctors and researchers in recent years. It has been urged that advice given at the first ante-natal appointment is simply too late — most miscarriages have already happened. In pregnancies that continue, all the major organs will be formed. The spine, for instance, is formed very early in pregnancy, when a sheet of cells folds into a tube. This major reorganization in the embryo takes place at between four and six weeks of pregnancy, before most women would know they were pregnant. A dietician who sees the mother at her first ante-natal appointment may give her good advice about eating more fresh green vegetables, but for babies with spina bifida it is tragically too late.

The argument for pre-conception care has been put most strongly in this country by the charity Foresight. Foresight are starting to open clinics where couples planning pregnancy are given expert advice. If you attend such a clinic, the doctor will look at your nutritional status, assess the levels of toxins such as lead in your body, test you for allergic reactions, and give you advice geared to your own individual needs. This service is very comprehensive but, as it is private, it is of course beyond many people's financial means. Pre-conception counselling has recently become available in some centres on the NHS. There is an urgent need for it to be made more widely available.

The chances are that, unless you seek it out deliberately and can afford to pay, you will not be given even the most basic pre-conception counselling. This is why this chapter includes suggestions that you and your partner can follow for yourselves to prepare for the next pregnancy. These strategies can form the basis of your own 'training programme' for pregnancy. Put like this, it may all sound rather strenuous, but for many women after miscarriage, the discipline is welcome. Many of us feel that we would do almost anything to reduce the chances of miscarrying again.

The analogy with sport can be pushed too far, of course. Fran would not have got beyond the first mile or two of that marathon if she had not put in some training, but women on very poor diets, exposed to toxic hazards and with no medical care, do still produce perfectly healthy babies. The woman who has already had one or more miscarriages would seem to be particularly well advised to prepare for her next pregnancy. Yet if she has already had three miscarriages, she still has a two out of three chance of having a healthy baby next time — even if she does nothing at all to prepare.

Sadly, of course, even if you do everything right, you may still have another miscarriage. Pregnancy is a gamble. But even with gambling, there may be ways of improving your chances. A man who puts money on the horses will be much more likely to win if he studies form. And with pregnancy, too, there are ways to give yourself a better chance of winning through.

WHAT IS A GOOD DIET?

A browse through old cookery books shows just how much our ideas about good food have changed. According to food writers of the fifties, the most nourishing foods were the bland white ones. Invalids were given steamed fish in white sauce and milk puddings. Milk was seen as an ideal food, easily digested and full of goodness. 'White' meant nourishing, healing, free of dangerous impurities. Nowadays it is not white but brown foods that have that aura of virtue. Health-conscious people choose brown bread, brown rice, muesli and bran. Brown food has come to embody a new set of values, now seen as desirable in food — brown is natural, wholesome, brimful of health-giving nutrients, just like great-grandmother used to make, just like people eat in healthy peasant societies. Values that fit brown flour or brown rice well enough, but what about the preference for brown sugar — identical to white in food value, except that it has a minute amount of extra iron? Or the widespread belief that brown eggs are somehow better than white, although they differ only in colour?

Giving things up is another preoccupation. Slimming is one aspect of giving things up. Anorexic women remain the fashionable ideal, and it is said that 50 per cent of women at any one time are on a slimming diet. Giving things up also means avoiding particular foods. Magazines carry articles informing us that certain foods are bad for us and best avoided. Milk and eggs, formerly thought 'good', are high on the list of foods to be deplored. The discovery of the role of food allergy in illness has led to another variation on the theme. People may mistakenly diagnose themselves as having allergic reactions and give up foods which would be good for them. Audrey Eyton's book, *The F-Plan Diet*, published in 1982, described how to get very thin by eating lots of bran. It is a perfect blend of these two preoccupations — brown food and giving things up. No wonder it was a best-seller.

Of course some of the advice we are given is based on hard evidence. Certain brown foods are indeed more nourishing than their white equivalents and, for one vulnerable group of people, giving up some dairy produce may indeed reduce the risk of heart disease. However there are question marks over a number of current food fashions. Recently, for instance, there has been concern about the increased incidence of osteoporosis, a weakening of the bones in women after menopause. Osteoporosis may be caused by low calcium intake, and if you eat a lot of bran and raw vegetables — foods seen as 'healthy' — you will absorb less calcium and may increase your chances of suffering from this painful complaint.

Am I right, too, in suspecting that there is a sexist bias in current food advice? A good diet for a woman who is conceiving, bearing and breastfeeding a child may be very different from a good diet for a man of the same age with a sedentary job. A low fat vegetarian diet may be ideal for him, and lower his risk of having a heart attack. The woman, on the other hand, needs more protein, and if she diets too rigorously, and her fat-to-body ratio drops below a certain point, she will become infertile as she will stop ovulating. She is also much more likely than the man to become deficient in elements like iron and zinc, of which meat is a rich source. Perhaps he should nibble the cottage cheese salad, while she has lunch at the local steak house.

HEALTHY EATING TO PREPARE FOR PREGNANCY

1. Eat a well-balanced diet.
Try to eat foods from each of these groups every day:
(a) Grains: bread, rice, breakfast cereal, crispbread, etc.
    These will provide you with carbohydrates, essential B vitamins, and some protein.
(b) Vegetables and fruit
    If you cannot afford much fruit, eat plenty of fresh vegetables. Try especially to eat leafy vegetables such as broccoli, brussels sprouts, cabbage, dark leafy lettuce, endive, watercress. These all contain folic acid which is an essential nutrient in pregnancy.
(c) Meat, fish and eggs
    These are all good sources of protein. If you are vegetarian, then you will get your protein from alternative sources, such as pulses, grains and nuts in combination.
(d) Dairy products: milk, cheese, yoghurt
    These provide calcium and fat. Whole milk is preferable to skimmed.

2. Eat 'natural' food.
When food is processed, essential nutrients are lost, so choose food that is in a state as close as possible to the way it grew.

Choose wholemeal bread, brown rice and whole breakfast cereals. As far as possible, eat vegetables and fruit fresh rather than canned or frozen, and where appropriate eat vegetables and fruit with the peel on, well-washed.

3. Eat a wide variety of foods.
A good diet for pregnancy is not about deprivation. The principle is not to give things up, but rather to add new foods to your diet. Eat lots of different kinds of fruit and vegetables, try different cuts of meat, including liver and kidneys, alternative sources of protein like nuts and pulses, lots of fish including the oily ones like sardines, other grains as well as wheat — brown rice, oats, barley.

4. Make sure you are eating enough protein.
Protein is the basic building material of life and this is what the baby will need to grow. Protein quality depends on how much a food contains of each of the basic elements of protein, known as amino acids. All the amino acids occur in perfect combination in any single meat, fish or dairy food. Vegetable foods also contain amino acids, but no single one of them contains all the essential amino acids. So if you do not eat meat or fish, you must eat foods which contain complementary amino acids together, at the same meal. You can get complete proteins by eating, for instance, a grain and a pulse (eg butter beans and rice), a grain and a dairy product (eg macaroni cheese), a grain and a nut (eg a nut loaf made with breadcrumbs).

If you are vegetarian, and especially if you are vegan, you will need to take extra care with your diet. In her book *What Every Pregnant Woman Should Know*, Gail Sforza Brewer comments, 'Absolute vegetarians who use no animal protein in their diets must be extremely careful in planning their pregnancy diets ... A wiser course is to suspend absolute vegetarian diets during pregnancy and nursing. At the very least, they should be modified to include eggs and milk products. An absolute vegetarian diet that may sustain a nonpregnant woman will not suffice for pregnancy.' Her doubts about vegetarian and vegan diets in pregnancy are echoed by a number of other writers on nutrition. If you are vegetarian out of preference rather than principle, you might consider eating meat before and during pregnancy, and returning to your preferred diet once the baby is born.

You may eat little meat, not out of principle, but because you cannot afford it. Eating well on a low income takes great ingenuity. One way of boosting your protein intake is to combine small quantities of the cheaper cuts of meat with pulses or grains, for instance in casserole dishes.

Remember that you need carbohydrate to use protein. If your carbohydrate intake is too low, your body will simply burn the protein as energy.

5. Eat to appetite.

Do not try to lose weight when you are trying to get pregnant. Women who are underweight, may stop ovulating and be unable to conceive. Women who are pregnant and who go on strict diets, often in response to ill-judged medical advice, may be putting themselves and their babies at risk. Dieting in pregnancy increases the risks of toxaemia for the mother and low birth-weight for the baby, and possibly other complications as well. But if your partner is very obese, perhaps he should try to lose some weight. Obesity in men can lead to low sperm production.

6. Use a water filter.

A water filter will take most of the heavy metals, like lead and copper and also other pollutants, out of your water supply. The most widely available one is a jug with a charcoal filter and is on sale in many health food shops. If you do use a water filter, you must remember to change the filter cartridge regularly, about once a month, because if the cartridge becomes so saturated that it stops working, all the pollutants will be washed back into the water.

7. Take vitamin and mineral supplements.

Supplements specially formulated for pregnant women are preferable. When you are trying to conceive and during pregnancy, you should avoid so-called 'mega-doses' of any vitamin, including the widely available 1 gram Vitamin C tablets that many people now take for colds or flu. Foresight have had two supplements formulated for pregnant women, one containing vitamins and one containing minerals. You should be able to get these from well-stocked health food shops, or you can get them direct from Foresight 'Vitamin Service' (see Useful Addresses). You could take them for a month before you start to try and conceive, and throughout pregnancy, or at least for the first three months of pregnancy when the baby is most vulnerable.

If you would prefer not to take a complete supplement, consider at least taking a folic acid supplement, as research suggests that folic acid may protect against spina bifida and spina bifida may account for a significant proportion of miscarriages. You can ask your doctor to prescribe folic acid, or you can buy it over the counter in the larger health food shops.

If you are of Asian origin, you may need some extra vitamin D. Fatty fish, such as mackerel, pilchards and herrings, are good sources of vitamin D. Milk, eggs, cheese and butter also contain some vitamin D. However, it may be worth taking a supplement.

8. Restrict smoking and alcohol.

Two or three weeks into pregnancy, many women lose their appetite for alcohol. But the baby is vulnerable from the very beginning. So when you are trying to conceive, you should ideally avoid alcohol altogether. Your partner, too, should keep his alcohol intake down when you are trying to conceive.

You can get advice on giving up smoking from ASH, Action on Smoking and Health (see Useful Addresses). If you cannot give up, at least try to cut down, and eat the best diet you possibly can. You could also take vitamin and mineral supplements, preferably the sort that are formulated for pregnancy.

A good diet is of course not the whole answer to the problem of miscarriage, but sometimes diet does seem to be the key to success. Fiona had one pregnancy with toxaemia and a low birth-weight baby, then she had three miscarriages. 'We even went so far as to consider adopting a baby,' she said.

> Then I discovered what was wrong. I discovered Adelle Davis or at least her book, called simply *Let's Have Healthy Children*. It's all in Adelle's book, right from before the woman conceives, through the pregnancy and all the problems, large and small, and right up until the child is 12 years old. ... I went on to have a second baby, a boy, no toxaemia, no high blood pressure and no haemorrhage. The baby was a good weight, 7½ lbs, born exactly on time. I had a fourth miscarriage because I wasn't watching my protein intake, but with my third live pregnancy, another beautiful girl, I found I could even control my blood pressure.

SOURCES

Gail Sforza Brewer with Tom Brewer, *What Every Pregnant Woman Should Know*, Penguin, Harmondsworth, 1985
Literature published by Foresight, including 'Guidelines For Future Parents'

Barbara Pickard, *Eating Well For A Healthy Pregnancy*,
Sheldon, London, 1984

REFERENCES

1. Barbara Pickard, 'Preconception care', *Journal of Obstetrics and Gynaecology*, 4 (suppl. 1), 1984, S34-S43
2. World Health Organization, *Social and Biological Effects on Perinatal Mortality*, vol. 1, 1978
3. Barbara Pickard, in an article for the Miscarriage Association
4. Brewer, *op cit*, p. 132

11.
THE NEXT PREGNANCY

One for sorrow,
Two for joy,
Three for a girl,
Four for a boy.

At the start of my last pregnancy — the one that worked — we
were on holiday in Crete. I found myself suddenly revolted by
the smells of herbs and wine and olive oil that I'd loved before,
and I knew then I must be pregnant. Immediately I became
obsessed with the possibility of miscarriage. As I sat at the back
of a rickety old Greek bus, I felt every jolt as a threat to the
baby inside me. In the air-conditioned atmosphere on the plane,
away from the smells of Greek food, I started to feel less sick. I
told my husband, 'I'm going to have a miscarriage, I don't feel
pregnant any more.' That time he believed me. The eighth or
ninth time I made the same announcement he didn't take it
quite as seriously.

Being convinced it was going to happen was a way of keeping
on the right side of Fate. Flickerings of hope were ruthlessly
suppressed. There was a crazy unconscious logic to it — if I
don't allow myself to hope, even for a moment, then perhaps I
will be all right, but if I allow myself to dream about the baby
then I'm sure to miscarry. Vigilance was part of it too. I studied
my body for signs that pregnancy symptoms were fading, I was
always looking for that ominous pink stain.

As I passed the points at which I had miscarried before, I felt
a little better, but when at 14 weeks I went for a scan, I felt like
a fraud. I was convinced that once they looked at my womb,
they would find that there was nothing there. And I certainly
did not let myself lust after soft white woolly things in the
Mothercare window. I would not buy anything for the baby. I
told my friends I did not like baby clothes and half the time I
believed this fiction.

Time after time, I convinced myself that the baby had died, only to be reassured by a comforting wriggle against the wall of my stomach. When I was told, at 28 weeks, that the baby was small for dates, it felt like a confirmation of what I had always believed — of course, I couldn't have a normal healthy baby like other women. When she was finally placed on my stomach, it took me a while to register that it was a girl — I was so amazed that she was alive.

It sounds bizarre, but I know that my feelings and responses are shared by many women who have miscarried in the past when they become pregnant again. Pregnancy after miscarriage is far from being the time of blooming contentment suggested in the advertisements in the baby magazines. Many women behave like I did, weaving elaborate webs of superstition and denial, to try to protect themselves from the pain of loss.

HOW TO RELAX

'Don't worry,' say friends and relatives. They may even hint that all this anxiety is bad for the baby. Their advice is no help to you. You cannot control anxiety by an act of will, and if you try to, you find yourself in an Alice-in-Wonderland world where you worry about worrying, and there seems to be no escape.

But there are certain things you can do that will help you cope. By practising relaxation on a regular basis, you can make yourself feel more peaceful, and take time out from your worries.

For deep relaxation, you need to lie down somewhere warm and quiet, and make yourself as comfortable as possible. Make sure you will not be disturbed.

If you own or can borrow a cassette player, you could use a relaxation tape. These tapes are widely available, for instance in health food shops, and by post via the small advertisements in health magazines. Relaxation for Living (see Useful Addresses) is an organization which provides particularly good tapes and cassettes for learning to relax at home.

If you cannot listen to a tape, then you can take yourself through a relaxation sequence. This is a little more effort than using a tape. The principle of relaxation is to tense deliberately and then let go. Concentrate on one set of muscles in the body, tighten them, clenching them as tightly as you can, then let them flop. Work through your body, concentrating on one set of muscles at a time. Start with your feet and work upwards, tensing and then letting go the muscles of your legs, stomach, back, and arms, and then on to the neck and shoulders and the muscles of the face. Repeat this sequence three times.

Once your body is thoroughly relaxed, you can use a technique borrowed from meditation to clear your mind of thoughts and worries. In meditation you attempt to create a peaceful place inside yourself by concentrating on one thing. The 'one thing' might be your breath. Breathing deeply and slowly and gently, without forcing, count your breaths up to four over and over again, saying the number inside your head on the out-breath. Or the 'one thing' might be a mantra. A mantra is simply one word or several words that you say slowly over and over again in your head. Some mantras are taken from religious practice — for instance 'om', pronounced 'oh-m'. Or you can use a word or several words that have a special meaning for you, such as 'peace'.

Practising deep relaxation on a daily basis can make you feel stronger and better able to cope. If you go through a relaxation sequence regularly, you will start to be more relaxed whatever you are doing, as you learn to recognize the signs of tension in your body and to let go. Regular meditation (20 minutes twice a day) has also been proved to keep blood pressure down in pregnancy.[1] These benefits are worthwhile in themselves. What may at first seem more surprising is that there may be benefits for the baby as well. I have described a study that suggested that 'optimal psychological support' is helpful to women who have suffered recurrent miscarriages. It has been suggested that this is because blood flow to the womb may be increased when the woman relaxes. Some centres that specialize in treating women who have suffered recurrent miscarriages are now using relaxation tapes as part of their treatment. Learning these techniques, then, may not only help you cope with the worry about miscarriage, but may also make it a little less likely to happen.

'NEVER MIND THE MILK, WHEN'S THE LOVING COMING IN?'

So there he or she is — your gorgeous perfect baby, slippery and creamy white, snuffling on your stomach, taking those first breaths, wonderfully alive, the apple of your eye. 'I have never seen a thing more clear,' wrote poet Sylvia Plath of this moment. Your joy is mixed a little with poignancy, perhaps — thoughts too of the baby you lost. But overwhelmingly a time for delight — a moment to cry with happiness instead of pain. And instantly you fall in love.

That is how it happens for many women — the love, the vividness, the tears of happiness. But it may be as well to know

151

that for women who have had miscarriages in the past, it is not always like that. This is Clara's story:

David was born after a worried but basically uneventful pregnancy, apart from a cervical stitch inserted before I became pregnant and hormone treatment. He was the baby I and my husband had longed for for nearly three years, but I simply didn't want him. I was not suffering from typical post-natal depression, and I cuddled him and fed him and did all the right things but I really didn't love him. He was a nuisance and a frustration (in the way all babies can be!) but there wasn't that compensating, overwhelming love.

Everyone was so delighted for us, but I felt very alone and so guilty for not being happy with the baby we had longed for. He was the fulfilment of a lifetime's longing, and I didn't want him. And feeling ungrateful and guilty just made it all worse. My question was 'Never mind the milk, when's the love coming in?'

So often the love flows easily. 'Why not for me?' Clara wondered. 'Anti-climax after waiting so long? The usual post-natal hormone swings and upheaval of a new baby compounded by disappointment at not feeling a surge of love?' How distressing to have wanted this tiny creature so much, and to have gone through so much for this moment, and then to feel indifferent, even to feel that you do not want this yearned-for baby.

Teresa Kewley, who wrote an account of her miscarriage in *Spare Rib*, had a similar experience. Teresa puts a different interpretation on it. After her second miscarriage, she said, 'Pregnancy became an obsession. I had to get pregnant. I didn't even see the end product, the baby, in my mind. I just needed to be able to say "I'm pregnant." In fact when I finally did get pregnant with my daughter I was very upset when she was born because I was no longer pregnant! I rejected her and didn't want to know her at all for a few days while I got over my resentment with the pregnancy being over.'

A slow start to the flowering of love for their babies seems to be quite common among women who have had miscarriages in the past. Clara and Teresa suggest some reasons for this: a sense of anti-climax when the moment you have yearned for so much finally arrives, resentment at the ending of the treasured state of pregnancy, the effects of the hormonal upsets after birth. I wonder, too, about the cost of all those months when you perhaps tried not to hope too much, tried not to imagine the moment when your baby would be put in your arms, even tried to pretend you were not pregnant at all — all the strategies some of us adopt in pregnancy to try and soften the pain a little if we do miscarry. It is as though you shut off a part of yourself to protect yourself from pain, and it takes a while to open up again with the birth of your baby.

Of course, it is not always like that. Usually, however troubled a woman's reproductive history, that 'compensating, overwhelming love' flows easily from the beginning. But if it should be slow to come from you, it may help to know that it has been like that for other women, too, and that in time your feelings will change.

Clara said, 'It did come right. By the time he was a year old, I did feel that all-encompassing love we are led to expect, and it has grown and grown. He is the most wonderful little boy and nothing will ever change my love for him.'

SOURCES

Lawrence LeShan, *How To Meditate*, Turnstone Press, Wellingborough, 1974

REFERENCES

1.   B. Little *et al*, 'Treatment of hypertension in pregnancy by relaxation and biofeedback', *The Lancet*, 21 April 1984, p. 866

CONCLUSION

After the birth of her daughter, Judith said, 'I dreamt about the first lost baby, as a boy toddler — not a sad or happy dream, just matter-of-fact. I'll never forget him, but the extreme happiness now compensates.'

The birth of a child answers some of the questions that miscarriage poses: 'No, there is nothing wrong inside me.' 'No, I am not being punished for something wrong I did.' If the miscarriages filled you with doubts about your body, your femaleness, or your capacity to love, these doubts are resolved in the day-to-day challenges and miracles of bringing up your child. For Judith, the 'matter-of-fact' quality of her dream points to a kind of acceptance. The miscarriage happened and she does not want to forget it, but some of the sadness is cancelled out by the birth of her daughter.

No woman would deny that the birth of a child assuages much of the pain of miscarriage. Yet I wonder whether any of us ever reach a state of complete acceptance. Looking back years later, and often after the births of healthy children they adore, women still wonder why it had to happen. Laura asked, 'Can anyone tell me how to fully come to terms with miscarriage? I've accepted it, I suppose, and I know that compared to women who've had more than one miscarriage or who have no children at all I'm lucky. But the older I get, the more difficult I find it coming to terms with the injustice of it all.' Liz said, 'I don't have any answers to miscarriage. My three experiences were totally heartbreaking and I can't find any explanation or reason for them. I had to live through them and they will always be part of my life.' For those women for whom miscarriage is part of a pattern of infertility, the 'injustice of it all' will continue to be a source of intense distress and pain.

'I don't want to forget'. 'My miscarriages will always be part of my life.' These statements need to be made in a society which does want us to forget and which keeps quiet about the part that miscarriage plays in so many women's lives. Occasionally in the last few years that silence has been broken, by the media and in particular by women's magazines. Maybe society is ready to discard the miscarriage taboo and to bring this hidden grief out into the light of day.

USEFUL ADDRESSES

The Miscarriage Association
18 Stoneybrook Close
West Bretton
Wakefield WF4 4TP
Tel: 092 485 515
Information and support for women who have had miscarriages, and their families. Runs self-help groups throughout the country.

SANDS (Stillbirth and Neonatal Death Society)
Argyle House
29-31 Euston Road
London NW1 2SD
Tel: 01 833 2851/2
Offers support for newly bereaved parents whose babies died between 28 weeks of pregnancy and one month after birth. Runs local support groups.

CHILD
Farthings
Gaunts Road
Pawlett
Nr Bridgewater
Somerset
Tel: 0278 683595
Self-help for couples with infertility problems, and a miscarriage support line.

NAC (National Association for the Childless)
318 Summer Lane
Birmingham
Tel: 021 359 4887
Newsletter and regional groups

NCT (National Childbirth Trust)
9 Queensborough Terrace
London W2 3TB
Tel: 01 220 3833
Runs miscarriage support groups in some parts of the country.

CRUSE
Cruse House
126 Sheen Road
Richmond
Surrey
Tel: 01 940 4818
Counselling service for the bereaved.

SATFA (Support After Termination For Abnormality)
c/o 22 Upper Woburn Place
London WC1H 0EP
Tel: 01 388 1382.

TAMBA (Twins and Multiple Births Association)
292 Valley Road
Lillington
Leamington Spa CV32 7UE
Offers support where one twin dies and is miscarried.

Association for Spina Bifida and Hydrocephalus
c/o 22 Upper Woburn Place
London WC1 0EP
Tel: 01 388 1382
Support for couples offered termination after amniocentesis.

Foresight
The Old Vicarage
Church Lane
Godalming
Surrey GU8 5PN
Tel: 042879 4500
Has a wide range of booklets on pre-conception care, eg
Guidelines for Future Parents, £2.00 plus SAE. Will also supply
information about private preconception clinics.

Also **Foresight Vitamin Service**
Mrs P. Aschwarden
Dellrose Cottage
Littlewick Road
Lower Knaphill
Woking
Surrey GU21 2JU
Tel: 04867 88845
Will supply Foresight Vitamin and Mineral Supplements if you
cannot obtain them locally.

VDU Workers' Rights Campaign
City Centre
32-35 Featherstone Street
London EC1
Tel: 01 608 1388
Information and advice for VDU operators.

ASH (Action on Smoking and Health)
5-11 Mortimer Street
London W1N 7RH
Tel: 01 637 9843
Information on hazards of smoking and advice on how to give
up.

Relaxation for Living
29 Burwood Park Road
Walton-on-Thames
Surrey KY12 5LH
Tel: 0932 227826
Supply relaxation tapes and cassettes.